Standing Tai Chi for Seniors Over 60

Easy Home Exercises to Improve Balance, Ease Joint Pain, and Sharpen Mental Clarity — Illustrated 28-Day Workout Program, 10 Mins Daily, No Equipment Needed

Liuhe Chen

Disclaimer

This book is intended for general informational and educational purposes only. The exercises and guidance contained in this publication are not a substitute for professional medical advice, diagnosis, or treatment. Always consult your physician or qualified healthcare provider before beginning any new exercise program, particularly if you have a pre-existing medical condition, recent injury, or surgery.

The author and publisher assume no responsibility for any injury, loss, or damage incurred as a result of the use or application of information contained in this book.

Table of Contents

A Note from the Author 1

Before You Begin 3

Chapter 1 6

Your Body at 60 – What's True and What Isn't 6

   Three Things That Actually Change After 60 6

   The Pain-Avoidance Trap 7

   Why Standing Practice Is Different 9

   Balance, Joints, and a Clearer Mind 11

Chapter 2 13

What Tai Chi Does to the Body and Brain 13

   How Slow Standing Movement Rebuilds Joint Health 13

   Stress and Why Your Mind Feels Foggy 14

   Proprioception – The Sense You Didn't Know You Were Losing 15

   What 10 Minutes Daily Changes Over 28 Days 17

Chapter 3 19

Know Your Body First 19

   What Your Joints Are, Why They Hurt, What Helps 19

   The Best Time to Practice and Why 20

   Knees, Hips, and Shoulders 21

   Reading Your Body's Signals During Practice 23

   Your Day One Self-Assessment 24

Chapter 4 26

The Standing Forms 26

   The Nine Core Standing Forms 26

      Form 1: Opening Form 26

      Form 2: Ward Off 28

      Form 3: Roll Back and Press 30

      Form 4: White Crane Spreads Wings 33

      Form 5: Repulse the Monkey 35

      Form 6: Fair Lady Works the Shuttles 37

      Form 7: Golden Rooster Stands on One Leg 39

Form 8: Turn and Kick 40

Form 9: Closing and Return 42

Breath Timing for Every Movement 44

Common Mistakes and How to Spot Them 44

Mistake 1: Locked Knees 45

Mistake 2: Raised Shoulders 46

Mistake 3: Gaze Directed at the Feet 47

Mistake 4: Holding the Breath 49

Mistake 5: Weight Not Fully Transferred 50

Mistake 6: Arms and Legs Moving Out of Coordination 51

Balance Builders 52

Balance Builder 1: Tandem Stand 52

Balance Builder 2: Heel Raise with Eyes Closed 54

Balance Builder 3: Lateral Weight Shift 55

Balance Builder 4: Single-Leg Reach 56

Chapter 5 59

The 28-Day Program 59

Week 1 – Grounded and Still 59

Learning to Stand Before You Move 63

Managing Stiffness in the First Week 63

Week 2 – Open the Joints 63

Knees, Hips, and Shoulders Getting Their Turn 67

Week 3 – Sharpen the Mind...67

Focus, Coordination, and the Mind-Body Shift 71

Week 4 – Stand Tall, Stay Sharp 71

End of Week Four: Full Body and Mind Review...75

Chapter 6 76

Sleep, Rest, and the Recovery Loop..76

Why Recovery Is Half the Practice...76

How Tai Chi Changes Sleep Quality After 60 77

What Happens to Joints During Sleep...78

What Happens to Balance During Rest 79

What Happens to Mental Clarity During Sleep 80

The Morning Window – Your Most Powerful 10 Minutes 80

Chapter 7 82

Living in a Sharper, Steadier Body 82

Applying the Forms to Daily Life At Home 82

Reaching, Bending, and Lifting Without Pain 83

Mental Sharpness Beyond the Practice.................................84

Daily Habits That Lock In the Gains.....................................85

Chapter 8 87

After Day 28 87

Three Honest Questions to Ask Yourself 87

When to Progress, When to Repeat, When to Rest 88

Joint Pain That Didn't Shift – What to Do Next.................89

Turning 28 Days Into a Lifelong Rhythm 90

Conclusion..93

About The Author...95

A Note from the Author

Three things brought you here. Your balance may feel less certain than it used to. Your joints may wake up stiff or ache through the afternoon. Your thinking may feel slower or foggier than it did a decade ago. You may be dealing with one of these things or all three simultaneously. Any of them is enough of a reason to start this program.

I want to explain right at the beginning why these three things are addressed in a single book and a single practice, and why that is not a marketing convenience but an accurate account of how the body actually works.

Balance, joint pain, and cognitive clarity are not separate problems with separate solutions. They run on the same underlying systems: the nervous system, the hormonal environment, and the feedback loops between movement and the brain. When balance deteriorates, the fear of falling produces chronic low-level tension that stiffens the very joints that are already under stress. When joints are chronically inflamed, the resulting pain disrupts sleep, and disrupted sleep elevates cortisol, and elevated cortisol impairs the kind of clear, responsive thinking that daily life requires. The problems compound each other. That is why so many people over sixty find that everything seems to be getting harder at the same time, even when no single diagnosis explains all of it.

Tai Chi addresses this system, not the individual symptoms. The slow, controlled movement lubricates joints through deliberate weight-shifting and rotation. The breath coordination lowers cortisol, which reduces both joint inflammation and cognitive fog. The mental focus required to move through precise sequential forms activates the prefrontal cortex in ways that are specific and measurable. These are not separate effects. They happen in the same ten-minute session, in the same body, simultaneously.

I have taught standing Tai Chi to older adults for a long time. The first thing most people notice is not what they expected. They expected balance or joint relief. What they usually notice first, within ten days to two weeks, is that they sleep better. That they wake up less stiff. That the morning transition from bed to bathroom to kitchen feels easier than it did before the practice. This is not a coincidence. The cortisol reduction from daily deliberate movement is the mechanism, and sleep is the first place most people feel it.

The joint relief tends to come next, around the three-week mark, as the synovial fluid production that slow movement stimulates begins to make a consistent difference. The balance improvements, which are actually the most substantial and durable of the three benefits, take the full twenty-eight days and beyond to appear at their fullest, because proprioceptive retraining is a neural process, and neural processes consolidate slowly and permanently.

The mental clarity shift is the hardest to measure and the most commonly reported by people who have stayed with the practice past the first month. They describe it as becoming more present, more focused during ordinary tasks, quicker to find words, less fatigued by cognitive demands. The neurological explanation for this is in Chapter Two. I mention it here because it is real, and because it tends to be the benefit that surprises people most.

This program is ten minutes a day. It requires a clear floor space about the size of a yoga mat, a sturdy chair nearby, and flat shoes or bare feet. Nothing else. You do not need to know anything about Tai Chi before you begin. You need to be willing to stand still and pay attention for ten minutes each morning. That is the entire requirement.

Start at Chapter Three before Day 1. Take the three assessments. They are short and they will make the Day 28 progress review more honest and more useful. Then come to Chapter Five with the forms from Chapter Four already read, if not memorized. The program will teach the forms as it goes.

Begin simply. Do not rush the opening weeks. The practice is a long one, and these first ten minutes are the foundation of everything that follows.

Liuhe Chen

Before You Begin

A few things to settle before Day 1. They take less time to read than they will save you in the weeks ahead.

Medical Disclaimer

Please speak with your doctor before starting this program if any of the following apply: you have experienced a fall in the past twelve months; you have been diagnosed with a vestibular disorder, severe osteoporosis, or Parkinson's disease or another neurological condition affecting balance or coordination; you have had hip, knee, or shoulder surgery within the past six months; you have uncontrolled hypertension or a cardiac condition requiring supervised exercise; or you have been advised by a healthcare provider to avoid weight-bearing activity.

This program consists of slow, controlled standing movements performed within a small floor space with a chair available for support. It is among the gentlest categories of physical practice available to older adults. That said, standing movement involves balance demands, and balance demands carry some fall risk, particularly in the early weeks when the forms are unfamiliar. The risk is manageable with proper setup and attention. The setup instructions below address it directly.

If you experience dizziness, chest tightness, shortness of breath, or sharp pain in any joint during a session, stop. Sit in your chair. Rest. If symptoms persist, seek medical attention. Contact your physician before continuing the program.

What You Need

The space requirements are minimal. You need a floor area of approximately six by six feet that is clear of furniture, cables, and any tripping hazard. A non-slip surface is preferred. Thick carpet is not ideal for the balance forms in Week Three and Four; low-pile carpet or a smooth floor with flat shoes is better. If your available space is carpeted throughout, wear flat-soled shoes with good grip and practice close to a wall.

A sturdy chair is required. Not a desk chair on wheels, not a low soft armchair. A dining chair or kitchen chair with a stable base and a back you can grip if needed. Place it at the edge of your practice space within two steps of where you will stand. It does not need to be used. Knowing it is available is what allows the practice to be relaxed.

Wear flat shoes or practice in bare feet. Avoid thick-soled running shoes, which raise the center of gravity and reduce the ground feel the balance forms depend on. If you have orthotics, wear them with low-profile walking shoes.

That is the complete equipment list. No mat, no resistance bands, no props of any kind. The practice uses the body and the space. Both are already available to you.

How to Use This Book

Chapter One introduces the three-problem system this program addresses, balanced against a realistic account of what the practice can and cannot do. Read it before Day 1.

Chapter Two covers the science behind all three benefits: balance, joint health, and mental clarity. It provides the framework that makes the coaching notes in Chapter Five meaningful rather than arbitrary. Reading it is not required to follow the program, but it changes the quality of attention you bring to each session.

Chapter Three prepares your body and establishes the three baselines that the progress checks in Chapter Five measure against. Complete the Day One Self-Assessment before beginning the program. Without it, the progress checks at Day 14, Day 21, and Day 28 have no reference point.

Chapter Four is the form library. Every standing form in the 28-day program is written out in full here with step-by-step instructions and image prompts. Read through each form before it appears in Chapter Five. You do not need to memorize the forms before Day 1. You need to have seen each one at least once.

Chapter Five is the daily program. It is organized into four weekly phases, each with a distinct theme. Read the week overview at the beginning of each new week before the first session of that week.

Chapter Six covers sleep, rest, and recovery. This chapter is unique among Tai Chi books for seniors and addresses why recovery is not a passive period between sessions but an active part of the three-benefit system this practice delivers. Read it before Week Two begins.

Chapters Seven and Eight address daily life application and what comes after Day 28. Read them when they become relevant.

One important note about rest days. Two rest days are scheduled in each week of this program, on the days where the body most benefits from consolidation. Do not replace them with extra practice sessions. The rest days are where the proprioceptive, joint, and cognitive gains from the practice sessions become durable.

One practice note before you begin. The forms in this book move slowly. More slowly than feels natural. This is deliberate. The balance training, the joint lubrication, and the cognitive engagement that this practice produces all depend on the slow pace being maintained. If a form feels too easy at the Tai Chi pace, the instruction is not to move faster. It is to pay closer attention to what is happening inside the form at the pace it requires.

Chapter 1

Your Body at 60 – What's True and What Isn't

Sixty is a number that arrives with a set of assumptions attached. Some of them are accurate. Others have been accepted without examination. This chapter deals honestly with both.

Three Things That Actually Change After 60

The body after sixty is a body that has been in continuous use for six decades. Most of what changes with age changes gradually, and most of it is manageable with the right kind of attention. Some of what changes, though, is genuinely significant, and pretending otherwise does not help anyone.

The first significant change is proprioceptive decline. Proprioception is the nervous system's capacity to know where the body is in space without using the eyes. Every joint contains mechanoreceptors, sensory nerve endings that register pressure, position, and movement and relay that information to the brain in real time. After sixty, the density and responsiveness of these receptors begins to decrease. The brain receives a less detailed picture of where the limbs are and how the weight is distributed. The result is a subtle but consequential reduction in balance precision, particularly on uneven surfaces or during movement transitions.

This is not obvious from the outside. People with significantly reduced proprioception can appear to walk normally on familiar terrain in good conditions. The deficit shows up in specific situations: stepping off a curb onto an unexpected surface, standing on one leg to put on a shoe, turning quickly to respond to a sound. These are the moments where a body relying on less proprioceptive precision is vulnerable, and where falls are most likely to occur.

The second significant change is synovial fluid dynamics. The joints of the body, particularly the weight-bearing joints of the hips, knees, and ankles, are lubricated by synovial fluid. This fluid is produced by the synovial membrane that lines each joint cavity and it performs several functions simultaneously: it reduces friction between cartilage surfaces, delivers nutrients to the cartilage cells that have no direct blood supply, and carries away metabolic waste products. After sixty, synovial fluid production slows and its viscosity changes. The cartilage receives less nutrition, waste products accumulate more readily, and the friction between joint surfaces increases. The result is stiffness, particularly pronounced after periods of inactivity, and an escalating cycle of minor inflammation that becomes the background noise of daily life for many older adults.

The third significant change is the stress-cognition interaction. The brain after sixty produces and clears cortisol less efficiently than it did earlier in life. Cortisol is the primary stress hormone, and its effects on cognitive function are extensive: it impairs working memory, reduces processing speed, interferes with attention, and disrupts the overnight consolidation of memory and learning that happens during deep sleep. Chronic low-level cortisol elevation, which many older adults carry without identifying it as stress, is one of the most consistent drivers of the cognitive changes that feel like natural aging but are actually, at least in part, physiological responses to an endocrine system that is running hot.

These three changes are separate in mechanism but tightly interconnected in effect. This chapter traces those connections.

The Pain-Avoidance Trap

There is a pattern of adaptation to joint pain and balance uncertainty that is rational at the individual level and harmful at the systemic level. It unfolds in a recognizable sequence.

Joint discomfort during movement prompts the person to reduce the movements that cause or aggravate it. This is a sensible response to pain. The reduction in movement, however, reduces the circulation and synovial fluid production that the affected joint depends on. A joint that moves less produces less lubrication and receives less nutritional delivery to its cartilage. The pain that prompted the movement reduction tends to worsen rather than improve. More movement reduction follows.

Simultaneously, the reduction in general movement reduces the proprioceptive input the nervous system receives. The mechanoreceptors in the joints are stimulated by movement and pressure. A body that moves less gives them less to work with, and the neural pathways that carry proprioceptive information to the brain become less active. Reduced activity in these pathways is associated with further decline in proprioceptive acuity. The balance that was already less precise than it was at forty becomes less precise still.

The balance uncertainty that results from reduced proprioception produces a characteristic response: protective tension. The body braces. The muscles of the back, neck, and hips maintain a higher resting tone than is needed for the current activity, consuming energy and producing a fatigue that is disproportionate to the physical demand. This chronic muscular bracing is itself painful over time, adding a secondary layer of discomfort on top of the original joint pain that initiated the cycle.

The cognitive dimension of this cycle is the most overlooked component. Chronic pain is cognitively expensive. Managing pain requires continuous attention and emotional resources. The brain monitoring and modulating pain signals has fewer resources available for the tasks that require clear thinking: forming and retrieving memories, maintaining focus through complex tasks, processing new information efficiently. The cognitive symptoms that older adults attribute to aging are frequently, in significant part, the cognitive cost of managing ongoing pain in a body that has reduced its movement to protect itself.

There is also a social withdrawal pattern that compounds the physiological one. As movement becomes more cautious and more limited, the situations that feel manageable shrink. The walk to the end of the street, the visit to a neighbor, the trip to the market, each of these activities carries a balance and pain calculation that was previously automatic. When the calculation regularly comes out on the side of staying home, the person moves less, socializes less, and experiences the combined effects of reduced movement and reduced social engagement on both the body and the cognitive system. Isolation is independently associated with cognitive decline in older adults, and the movement restriction that comes from the pain-avoidance trap is one of the most consistent pathways into it.

Understanding the trap is not the same as escaping it. But it is the necessary first step, because the trap works partly through its invisibility. Each individual accommodation seems sensible. Only the accumulated pattern reveals the problem. Naming it clearly is what makes it possible to make deliberate choices about which accommodations are genuinely necessary and which ones can be walked back through careful, graduated practice.

Elevated cortisol compounds this further. The stress of pain, reduced mobility, and the fear of falling all drive cortisol production. Elevated cortisol stiffens joints by promoting pro-inflammatory cytokine activity. Stiff, inflamed joints are more painful. More pain produces more cortisol. The cycle closes.

The only sustainable intervention in this cycle is movement that is safe enough to be maintained despite the discomfort, specific enough to produce the joint lubrication and proprioceptive training that reverse the underlying changes, and cognitively engaging enough to interrupt the pain-attention loop and activate the prefrontal regulatory systems that modulate the stress response. Standing Tai Chi is specifically designed around those requirements. This is not an incidental coincidence. Tai Chi was developed and refined over centuries as a practice for older practitioners who could no longer use their bodies at high intensity but needed a practice that continued to develop their capacities rather than maintain them in comfortable decline.

Why Standing Practice Is Different

The distinction between standing Tai Chi and other forms of gentle exercise recommended for older adults is worth examining precisely, because the specific qualities that make Tai Chi effective for this population are not shared by the alternatives.

Walking provides cardiovascular benefit and some proprioceptive input through the heel strike. It does not require deliberate weight-shifting, does not involve the slow controlled rotation that lubricates the hip and shoulder joints specifically, and does not demand the sustained focused attention that produces the cognitive benefits this practice delivers. Walking is valuable and should not be discontinued. It is not a substitute.

Chair-based exercise removes the balance demand that is central to the proprioceptive training component. For individuals who genuinely cannot stand safely, seated practice is the appropriate starting point. But the balance training that standing Tai Chi delivers cannot be replicated in a chair. The brain learns to manage standing balance by managing standing balance, not by proxy.

Swimming and water aerobics are excellent for joint mobility and pain reduction, and for individuals with severe joint disease they may be the most appropriate primary exercise. The proprioceptive input from water exercise is reduced because water supports the body and removes the full-weight ground-contact signals that the mechanoreceptors in the ankles and feet depend on. The standing balance training that this program produces cannot be replicated in a pool.

Standing Tai Chi is distinct because it combines all three required elements simultaneously within a practice that is low-impact, low-risk, requires no equipment, can be done at home in ten minutes, and can be scaled from the beginning of balance impairment through to a lifelong practice for individuals who want to continue challenging themselves. No other common exercise recommendation for older adults checks all of these boxes. That is why this book exists.

The specific qualities that make standing Tai Chi uniquely effective are: the slow pace, which keeps the heart rate in the fat-oxidizing, cortisol-reducing range while keeping impact forces minimal; the deliberate weight-shifting between feet, which provides precisely the proprioceptive training that the mechanoreceptors need; the breath coordination, which activates the parasympathetic nervous system and reduces cortisol; and the sequential memorization and execution of the forms, which activates the working memory, spatial processing, and executive function circuits of the prefrontal cortex in a way that gentle exercise without motor complexity does not.

There is one additional quality worth naming: the practice is performed alone, at home, in a small space, with no requirement for a facility, a partner, a subscription, or a schedule negotiation. This reduces the barrier to daily practice to its absolute minimum. The single most consistent predictor of benefit from any exercise program for older adults is adherence. Standing Tai Chi at home eliminates most of the practical obstacles to adherence. It is done in the same space, at the same time, each morning, for ten minutes. That simplicity is a structural feature of the practice, not an afterthought.

It is also worth noting what happens to the forms themselves over weeks and months of regular practice. The learning curve is real, and the early sessions feel effortful in ways that the later ones do not. In the first week, the forms are sequences to be learned and remembered. By the fourth week, they begin to be experienced as patterns of sensation: the weight moving through the foot, the breath timing against the arm position, the specific quality of attention required to hold the balance in Golden Rooster. The practice becomes richer with familiarity rather than flatter. This is one of the characteristics that allows it to sustain engagement over years, something that simple repetitive exercises do not reliably do.

Balance, Joints, and a Clearer Mind

The three benefits of this practice are described separately in the chapter on science because the mechanisms are distinct. Here, before you read that chapter, it is worth understanding why they are actually a single system in practice, not three separate benefits.

Consider what happens during five minutes of Standing Tai Chi. The person stands with feet shoulder-width apart and shifts weight slowly from one foot to the other as the arms move through the form. The proprioceptors in the feet and ankles register every subtle change in pressure and position. The brain processes this proprioceptive input continuously and makes micro-adjustments to maintain balance. This is proprioceptive training, directly addressing the first significant change described above.

At the same time, the weight-shifting and joint rotation produce compressive and decompressive forces across the cartilage surfaces of the hips, knees, and ankles. These forces drive synovial fluid through the cartilage matrix, delivering nutrients and clearing waste. The joint is being lubricated and nourished while it moves. This is the joint health mechanism, directly addressing the second significant change.

At the same time, the person is tracking the sequential form, maintaining awareness of where the arms and weight are in relation to each other, and breathing in coordination with the movement. The working memory is holding the form sequence. The spatial processing system is managing the body's position. The prefrontal executive system is coordinating the breath with the movement and maintaining attention through the form. This is the cognitive engagement that distinguishes Tai Chi from simpler movement, directly addressing the third significant change.

None of these processes interferes with the others. They run simultaneously in the same body during the same ten minutes. This is why the improvements from this practice tend to appear across all three domains rather than in a single area, and why the improvements in one area tend to support the improvements in the others. Better balance produces less fear, which reduces cortisol, which improves cognitive clarity, which makes the form sequences easier to learn and maintain, which improves balance further. Better joint comfort reduces the cognitive overhead of pain management, freeing attention for the form work, which improves balance and reduces cortisol, which reduces joint inflammation. The three benefits are a system. The practice delivers the system.

It is also worth addressing what this practice is not claiming. It is not claiming to reverse joint damage that has already occurred, or to restore proprioceptive density that aging has reduced to its natural endpoint. What it claims is that the remaining capacity, whatever level it has reached in this particular body at this particular age, can be developed further and used more fully. The body at sixty-five with consistent deliberate practice is more capable than the body at sixty-five without it, not because the underlying processes of aging have been reversed, but because the available capacity has been systematically trained. That distinction matters. It is the difference between a promise that cannot be kept and a realistic outcome that the practice reliably delivers.

What 10 minutes a day can realistically do, over twenty-eight days, is begin this system running. The balance changes require the full program and will continue to develop beyond Day 28. The joint relief begins earlier, usually in the second or third week, as the synovial fluid production effect accumulates. The cognitive clarity shift is the most variable: some people notice it within two weeks, others after the first month. None of these timelines are fixed, and none of the outcomes are guaranteed. What is consistent across the research and across the experience of people who have completed this kind of practice is that something in all three areas improves for most people who show up for ten minutes daily and pay deliberate attention to what they are doing. That is the realistic promise. It is also a substantial one.

Chapter 2

What Tai Chi Does to the Body and Brain

The three benefits this practice delivers: better balance, less joint pain, clearer thinking. They are not incidental. They follow directly from specific physiological mechanisms. This chapter describes those mechanisms plainly. Understanding them changes how you practice.

How Slow Standing Movement Rebuilds Joint Health

Cartilage has no blood supply. This is an anatomical fact with significant consequences for how joints age and how they recover from stress. The nutrients that cartilage cells need to function, to maintain their matrix, and to resist degradation arrive not through capillaries but through a process called imbibition: the physical compression and decompression of the cartilage during movement drives synovial fluid through its matrix like water through a sponge. When you load a joint and then unload it, fluid is squeezed in and pushed out, delivering nutrients and clearing metabolic waste in the same mechanical action.

This means that joint health is directly dependent on movement. Not high-impact movement, not heavy loading, but regular, moderate, varied movement that compresses and decompresses the cartilage through its range. The cartilage of a joint that is not moved regularly receives less nutrition, accumulates more waste products, and degrades more quickly than cartilage that is regularly subjected to varied, moderate loading. The prescription for joint health is movement, and the movement that is most accessible, most consistent, and most appropriate for older adults with existing joint concerns is slow, controlled, weight-bearing movement.

Slow standing Tai Chi provides this in a specific form. The weight-shifting from foot to foot that runs through every standing form compresses and decompresses the cartilage of the ankles, knees, and hips in a continuous, rhythmic sequence. The rotational movements of the forms add torsional forces that the simple up-and-down loading of walking does not provide, lubricating the hip and shoulder joints in directions that ordinary ambulation leaves unaddressed. The slow pace keeps the loading forces moderate, which means the cartilage is nourished without being subjected to the kind of impact that aggravates inflammation.

The synovial membrane that produces synovial fluid is stimulated by gentle movement to increase its output. In a joint that has been relatively immobilized, this output is reduced and the fluid that is present may be less viscous and less nutritionally complete than fluid in an active joint. Regular gentle movement restores synovial membrane function. The joint that was stiff and dry after a night of inactivity becomes more mobile and better lubricated as the morning practice proceeds. This is not metaphorical. It is the mechanical and biochemical sequence.

The cortisol connection to joint pain is the other half of this mechanism. Cortisol promotes the production of pro-inflammatory cytokines, signaling molecules that drive the inflammatory processes in joint tissue. Chronically elevated cortisol maintains a chronic low-grade inflammatory environment in the joints that produces stiffness and pain even in the absence of structural damage. The cortisol reduction that regular slow Tai Chi practice produces through breath coordination and parasympathetic activation directly reduces this inflammatory signaling. The joint that was hurting partly because of cortisol-driven inflammation hurts less after four weeks of practice in which cortisol has been consistently reduced.

Stress and Why Your Mind Feels Foggy

The prefrontal cortex is the region of the brain most associated with what we call clear thinking: the ability to hold information in mind while working with it, to suppress irrelevant information in favor of the currently relevant, to plan sequences of action, to modulate emotional responses. It is also the region most vulnerable to cortisol.

Glucocorticoid receptors, the molecular targets for cortisol, are highly concentrated in the prefrontal cortex and the hippocampus. When cortisol levels are elevated, these receptors are saturated. The prefrontal cortex operates less efficiently. Working memory capacity decreases. Processing speed decreases. The ability to suppress distracting thoughts decreases. The cognitive experience of this is exactly what older adults describe as brain fog: thoughts that are harder to retrieve, attention that is harder to sustain, tasks that seem to require more effort than they used to.

The hippocampus, the region most directly involved in forming new memories and consolidating them during sleep, is similarly affected. Chronic cortisol elevation reduces hippocampal volume over years and impairs the overnight memory consolidation process. This produces the specific pattern of memory difficulty that older adults most commonly report: things learned yesterday are harder to recall today, new names and new information take longer to stick, and the memory feels less reliable in general.

Tai Chi practice addresses this through two distinct mechanisms. The first is cortisol reduction. The breath coordination in the forms, specifically the slow, diaphragmatic, extended exhale that characterizes proper Tai Chi breathing, activates the vagus nerve and shifts the autonomic nervous system toward parasympathetic dominance. Heart rate variability increases. Cortisol levels drop. The prefrontal cortex and hippocampus operate in a lower-cortisol environment. Over the weeks of the program, this reduction becomes a sustained feature of the practitioner's baseline hormonal environment, not just a temporary effect during the session.

The second mechanism is direct cognitive training through the forms themselves. Learning and executing the sequential motor programs of Tai Chi forms requires sustained engagement of the working memory, the spatial processing system, and the attentional control networks of the prefrontal cortex. This is not trivial mental activity. Holding the form sequence in mind while coordinating breath and movement and maintaining balance is a genuine executive function demand. The neural circuits that support these functions are strengthened by regular use, and their strengthening transfers to other cognitive tasks. This is the mechanism behind the consistent finding that regular Tai Chi practice is associated with better performance on cognitive tests in older adults.

Proprioception – The Sense You Didn't Know You Were Losing

Proprioception operates below the level of consciousness. It does not produce perceptible sensations the way vision or hearing does. You do not feel your proprioceptive system working any more than you feel your digestive system processing a meal. You only notice proprioception when it fails: the missed step on the dark staircase, the stumble on an uneven surface that you did not see in time to prepare for, the wobble when you stand on one leg to pull on a sock.

The mechanoreceptors that provide proprioceptive input are specialized sensory nerve endings in the joint capsules, ligaments, and muscles. They respond to changes in joint angle, tension in the surrounding tissue, and rates of change of position. They relay this information to the spinal cord and the brain continuously during movement. The brain uses this proprioceptive input, combined with visual input and vestibular input from the inner ear, to construct its real-time map of where the body is in space.

After sixty, the density of these mechanoreceptors in key joints decreases. The neural signals they produce become slower and less precise. The brain's real-time map of body position becomes less detailed. This is proprioceptive decline, and it is a central mechanism in age-related fall risk. A body with reduced proprioceptive acuity is slower to register a balance perturbation and slower to initiate the corrective response. The window between the perturbation and the correction becomes longer, and in that longer window, falls happen.

The specific training that restores proprioceptive acuity is the one that challenges it: controlled balance demands that require the proprioceptive system to produce accurate, rapid information under conditions of managed uncertainty. Standing Tai Chi forms provide this in graduated doses. The single-weight forms, where the body's weight shifts fully onto one foot, challenge the ankle and hip mechanoreceptors specifically. The transitional forms, where the weight transfers from one foot to the other through a controlled arc, provide the changing-position signals that train the rate-of-change receptors. The slow pace is essential: fast movement allows momentum to carry the body through balance transitions without requiring the proprioceptive system to manage them. Slow movement requires every transition to be actively managed, making the training more specific and more effective.

The vestibular system, which provides balance input from the fluid and hair cells of the inner ear, also benefits from the forms. The head movements in several forms, particularly Cloud Hands, provide the vestibular system with deliberate movement challenges in a controlled setting. This is fundamentally different from the vestibular challenges of ordinary daily life, which arrive without warning and without the option to move slowly through them.

The integration of proprioceptive, vestibular, and visual balance inputs is processed in the cerebellum and the brainstem, which coordinate these three streams into a coherent real-time balance command. When proprioceptive input is degraded, the brain leans more heavily on the visual and vestibular streams. This compensatory shift works adequately in good lighting on familiar terrain. It fails in poor lighting, on unfamiliar surfaces, or when the head moves in a way that provides ambiguous vestibular information. Tai Chi training strengthens the proprioceptive stream specifically, reducing the reliance on compensation and providing a more robust, multi-source balance system. The practical result is a person who is steadier in the specific situations where steadiness matters most: the poorly lit hallway at night, the uneven parking lot, the unexpected nudge from a shopping cart.

What 10 Minutes Daily Changes Over 28 Days

The adaptation timeline for this practice is predictable in its general shape even though individual timing varies.

In the first week, the primary adaptation is neurological familiarity with the forms. The brain is building the motor programs for the movement sequences, which requires heavy engagement of the working memory and the procedural learning systems. This is cognitively effortful, and many people find the first week mentally tiring in proportion to the brief physical duration of the sessions. This is the prefrontal cortex doing significant work. It is not a sign that the program is too hard.

In the second week, the cortisol reduction from daily practice begins to compound. Individual sessions produced temporary cortisol drops in Week One. In Week Two, the baseline cortisol level begins to shift downward as the daily practice creates a consistent pattern of parasympathetic activation. Sleep quality typically improves in Week Two for this reason. Morning stiffness often begins to ease as the joint inflammation that cortisol was driving reduces.

In the third week, the proprioceptive training begins to produce perceptible balance improvements. The mechanoreceptors in the weight-bearing joints have received fourteen to twenty-one days of deliberate training stimulation. The neural pathways carrying their signals have become more active and more efficient. People begin to notice that standing on one leg feels more stable, that transitions between activities feel less uncertain, that the fear response to balance perturbations is less automatic.

In the fourth week, the three benefits begin to be felt as a connected whole rather than separately. Better sleep is supporting clearer thinking. Clearer thinking is making the form sequences easier to maintain with attention. Better balance is reducing the fear and protective tension that were driving joint stiffness. Reduced joint stiffness is allowing more complete execution of the forms, which deepens all three mechanisms simultaneously.

By Day 28, the practice has produced changes in synovial fluid production, baseline cortisol, and proprioceptive neural pathway efficiency that are structural rather than temporary. They persist as long as the practice continues. They build further as the practice continues. The twenty-eight days are not the program. They are the beginning of the practice. Everything that follows is built on this foundation.

The most honest summary of what ten minutes a day over twenty-eight days produces is this: a body and mind that are measurably different from where they started in three specific ways, with those changes pointing in the direction of continued improvement rather than plateau. The practice is not a treatment with a defined course. It is a new relationship between the person and their body, established through daily attention. Day 28 is where that relationship begins to feel settled. What happens from Day 29 onward is up to the practitioner. The chapters that follow are the tools for making it continue.

Chapter 3

Know Your Body First

The forms in Chapter Four ask things of the joints, the balance system, and the attention that daily life has not been asking recently. This chapter prepares all three before the first session begins.

What Your Joints Are, Why They Hurt, What Helps

A joint is where two bones meet. The surfaces of those bones are covered with articular cartilage, a dense, smooth tissue that allows the surfaces to glide against each other with minimal friction. The joint is enclosed in a fibrous capsule lined with the synovial membrane, which produces the synovial fluid that lubricates the joint and nourishes the cartilage. Ligaments bind the bones together, and tendons attach the surrounding muscles to the bones, providing the controlled force that moves the joint.

When any element of this system is disrupted, pain and restricted movement follow. Cartilage that has thinned from decades of use loses its cushioning function and exposes the underlying bone to forces it was not designed to absorb. Synovial fluid that has become less viscous from reduced movement fails to lubricate adequately. Ligaments that have stiffened from chronic tension or previous injury restrict the range of available motion. Muscles that have shortened from prolonged sitting generate uneven forces across the joint surfaces, accelerating wear.

What helps is specific. Rest helps acute inflammation but worsens chronic stiffness by reducing the movement that produces synovial fluid and maintains cartilage nutrition. Anti-inflammatory medication reduces the pain signal but does not address the underlying mechanical causes. Deliberate, gentle, varied movement through the joint's available range restores synovial fluid distribution, provides the compressive stimulus that nourishes cartilage, and maintains the muscle balance that keeps joint forces even. This is what the standing forms in this program do, specifically and systematically, for the joints of the ankles, knees, hips, and shoulders.

The Best Time to Practice and Why

Morning stiffness is the experience of joints that feel thicker, less mobile, and more resistant to movement in the first minutes after waking. Its cause is the overnight accumulation of fluid and inflammatory proteins in the joint tissue during the reduced movement of sleep. The synovial fluid, which distributes through the joint during movement, settles and thickens overnight. The inflammatory products that the active immune response deposits in arthritic joints during sleep are present in higher concentrations in the morning than at any other time.

The fact that morning is often the most uncomfortable time to move is also, perhaps counterintuitively, one of the best times to practice. Morning practice catches the joint at the point of maximum stiffness, when the therapeutic benefit of deliberate movement is most needed and most rapid in effect. The ten minutes of standing forms, beginning with the Opening Form and its deliberate weight-shifting, drives synovial fluid back through the joint surfaces and accelerates the clearance of the inflammatory accumulation. Most people who practice consistently in the morning report that the stiffness resolves thirty to forty percent faster than on rest days.

The cortisol peak that occurs naturally in the first hour after waking, a physiological mechanism called the cortisol awakening response, is also relevant. This morning cortisol peak suppresses inflammation temporarily. Practicing at the tail end of this natural suppression window, roughly thirty to sixty minutes after waking, means the practice is occurring when the joint environment is biochemically most favorable. The forms then sustain the anti-inflammatory effect through the parasympathetic activation of their breath pattern, extending the window through the morning.

People who practice later in the day, after the cortisol awakening response has subsided and the day's demands have raised cortisol through different pathways, typically experience a smaller and less consistent joint effect. This does not mean evening practice is without value. It means morning practice is specifically advantaged for the joint outcomes this program prioritizes. If morning practice is genuinely impossible, late morning is the next best option. Afternoon is acceptable. Evening is better than no practice. Morning is best.

One practical note on the relationship between morning stiffness and session performance: the first two minutes of the Opening Form on a stiff morning will feel harder than the same two minutes after an easy morning. This is expected and correct. The point of morning practice is not that it is easy. The point is that the body that practices through the morning stiffness responds faster to the synovial stimulation of the forms than the body that waits until the stiffness resolves on its own.

Knees, Hips, and Shoulders

Before addressing each joint specifically, a general principle applies to all three: the pain signal in a chronically inflamed joint is not a reliable indicator of the actual structural state of the joint. Joints that feel severely painful are not always structurally worse than joints that feel only mildly uncomfortable. Pain is a neural signal that is amplified by fear, by the expectations that come from a bad history with a joint, and by the global cortisol environment. Reducing cortisol through the breath practice of the forms reduces the pain signal in all three joints simultaneously, independent of any structural change. This is why people sometimes report dramatic reductions in joint pain within two weeks, before structural changes could plausibly have occurred. The pain signal has reduced. The structure has not yet changed. Both matter.

Knees.

The knee is the most commonly symptomatic joint in this population and the one most likely to limit the early sessions. The standing forms involve continuous knee flexion: the fundamental position of all Tai Chi standing work requires a slight bend in both knees, and the weight-shifting forms require controlled single-knee loading through a range of flexion. For knees with significant osteoarthritis, the early sessions should use the minimum flexion that allows the form to be performed. Deeper knee bend is introduced gradually as the quadriceps strengthen and the synovial fluid production improves. Sharp pain localized to the knee joint during any form is the signal to reduce the bend angle. Aching that resolves within thirty minutes of the session is acceptable adaptation soreness.

A specific technique for managing knee discomfort during the forms is worth describing here. When the knee is painful at the depth of flexion the forms require, place both hands on the corresponding thigh and provide gentle downward pressure. This redistributes some of the quadriceps load through the hands and reduces the net load on the knee joint surface. It is a temporary accommodation that allows the form to continue while the quadriceps strengthen enough to manage the load independently. By Week Three most people who begin with this accommodation no longer need it.

Hips.

The hip is a ball-and-socket joint capable of movement in multiple planes. The standing forms address hip mobility in all these planes: the weight-shifting provides loading and unloading through the joint axis, the stepping forms provide rotation, and the forms that involve raising the leg, Golden Rooster specifically, provide hip flexion loading. The hip often responds more favorably to the forms than the knee, because the ball-and-socket design tolerates rotational forces well. Hip discomfort during the lateral stepping forms usually indicates tight hip flexors rather than joint pathology. Gentle hip flexor stretching before the session helps.

The hip flexor tightness that often accompanies hip joint pain deserves specific mention. Tight hip flexors pull the pelvis into anterior tilt, compressing the posterior hip joint capsule and altering the weight-bearing axis through the femoral head. The Ward Off and White Crane forms both require hip flexor lengthening through the standing position, and the deliberate neutral spine instruction that runs through all nine forms gradually releases chronic hip flexor tension. Most people with hip flexor tightness find the neutral spine position uncomfortable at first and then increasingly natural over the first two weeks. The discomfort is the flexors releasing.

Shoulders.

The shoulders are involved in every form as arm-movement joints, but they bear no body weight and are therefore less likely to be a limiting factor than the hips or knees. Shoulder restrictions most commonly manifest in the forms that require arm elevation above shoulder height. Fair Lady Works the Shuttles and the ward-off position of Opening Form both involve raised arms. If shoulder range of motion limits these forms, reduce the arm height until the shoulder is comfortable. Do not force elevation into pain. The shoulder range will increase as the surrounding rotator cuff muscles strengthen and the joint capsule loosens through repeated gentle movement.

Reading Your Body's Signals During Practice

Two categories of sensation arise during this practice, and distinguishing between them is essential. The inability to distinguish between them is the most common reason people stop a gentle practice that was actually helping them: they interpret productive discomfort as a warning signal and stop at precisely the point where the practice was beginning to produce meaningful change.

The first category is productive discomfort: the mild aching or fatigue in muscles that have been asked to work in a specific way they are not accustomed to, the joint warmth that accompanies the increase in synovial fluid circulation, the cognitive effort of holding a form sequence in working memory while managing balance. These sensations signal that the practice is working. They are appropriate and expected. They typically resolve within thirty minutes of the session and are absent or reduced within one to two weeks of consistent practice.

The second category is warning signals: sharp pain localized to a joint, pain that increases rather than levels off during the session, dizziness or significant breathlessness, pain that persists for hours after the session, or any sensation that feels qualitatively different from ordinary muscle effort. These are stop signals. Stop the form. Sit in the chair. Rest. If the sensation resolves within a few minutes, assess whether the form can be continued with reduced range or intensity. If it does not resolve, end the session and consult a healthcare provider before continuing the program.

A third signal specific to this program is the cognitive effort of the forms. Learning new motor sequences is effortful, and the mental fatigue of the first week is real. This is not a warning signal. It is the prefrontal cortex working hard to build new motor programs. By Week Two, the cognitive effort per session reduces as the forms become more familiar, and what was effortful becomes deliberate rather than labored.

The balance between productive effort and warning signals shifts over the course of the program. What was a warning signal in Week One, the wobble in Golden Rooster that required chair contact, may be a productive challenge by Week Three, managed without support. Reading the signals accurately requires comparing the current sensation to the current capacity rather than to a fixed standard. A sensation that was significant in Week One may be unremarkable in Week Three. The appropriate response evolves as the practice deepens.

Your Day One Self-Assessment

Take these three measurements before Day 1 of the program. Record them. They are the reference points for the progress checks at Days 14, 21, and 28.

Test One: Single-Leg Balance Hold.

1. Stand beside a sturdy chair with one hand available to touch it.
2. Shift your weight onto the left foot and lift the right foot just a few centimeters from the floor.

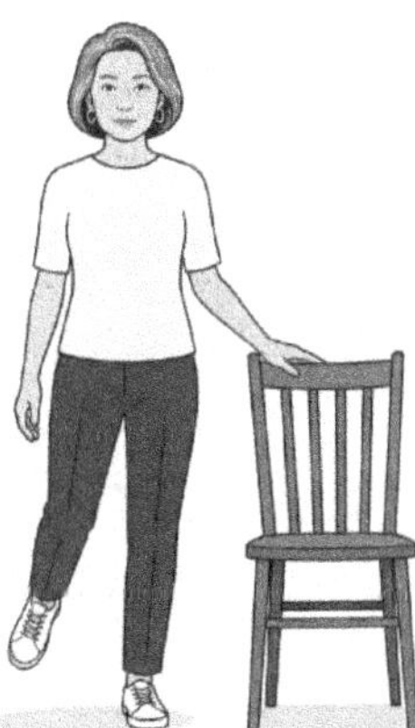

3. Release the chair. Count how many seconds you hold the position before needing to touch down or grab support.
4. Record the time. Repeat on the other side. Record both.
5. Note: if you cannot hold for five seconds without gripping, keep one fingertip lightly on the chair throughout the program's balance forms until the hold improves.

Test Two: Joint Stiffness Self-Rating.

On three consecutive mornings before Day 1, rate your joint stiffness immediately on waking, before getting up, on a scale of one to five. One means no stiffness. Five means significant stiffness that restricts movement for thirty minutes or more. Average the three readings. Record the average. This is your pre-program stiffness baseline.

Test Three: Three-Minute Focused Attention Test.

1. Sit in a chair with a clock or timer visible.

2. Choose a simple counting task: count backward from one hundred by threes. Alternatively, recite the alphabet and assign each letter a number, A equals 1, B equals 2, and so on.

3. Begin the task. Set a three-minute timer. Note how many times your attention drifts from the task to something else, requiring you to bring it back.

4. Record the number of attention lapses. This is your pre-program attention baseline. There is no right answer. It is simply your starting point.

Keep these three numbers. They will be referenced in the progress checks of Chapter Five. Without them, the checks have no meaningful reference.

Chapter 4

The Standing Forms

The movement library. Read through each form before the 28-day program. You need to have seen each one, not memorized it.

The Nine Core Standing Forms

Form 1: Opening Form

Establishes the fundamental standing alignment and breath pattern that all subsequent forms depend on.

1. Stand with feet shoulder-width apart, knees softly bent. Arms hang at sides, palms inward.

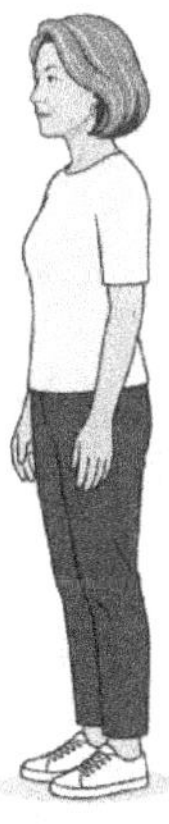

2. Lengthen through the crown of the head. Relax the shoulders away from the ears.

3. Inhale slowly. Allow both arms to float forward and upward to shoulder height, palms facing down.

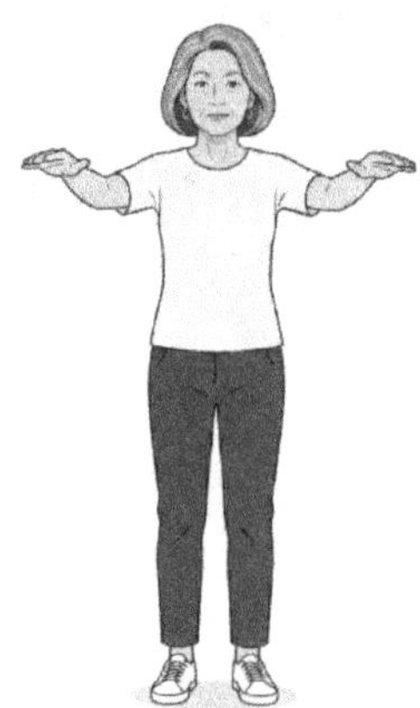

4. Exhale slowly. Lower the arms back to the sides.

5. Repeat three times. On the third lowering, let the arms settle. This completes the Opening Form.

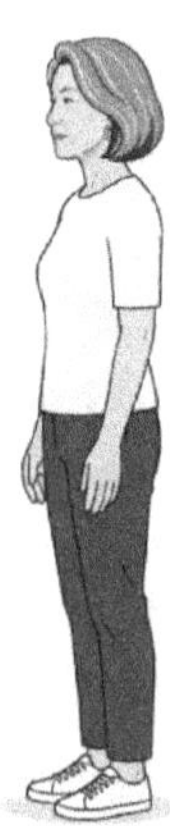

BREATHING: Inhale as the arms rise. Exhale as they lower. The breath leads the movement.

MIND NOTE: Track both palms simultaneously during the rise and lower, activating the spatial processing the practice builds.

JOINT NOTE: Initiates shoulder joint capsule movement and synovial fluid distribution before the more demanding forms begin.

BALANCE NOTE: Equal weight distribution throughout; any drift is proprioceptive feedback to observe, not forcefully correct.

WHAT THIS FORM DOES FOR YOU

Balance: Trains your body to stand evenly on both feet and use your breath to settle into stillness, which sharpens your postural awareness.

Joint Pain: Gently introduces movement to the shoulder joints before heavier forms begin, reducing the stiffness that comes from inactivity.

Mental Clarity: Focusing on both hands simultaneously activates the thinking and coordination parts of the brain, giving your mind a calm, deliberate point of entry into the practice.

SEATED MODIFICATION

Sit at the front of the chair, spine tall. Raise and lower the arms as described. Breath coordination is identical.

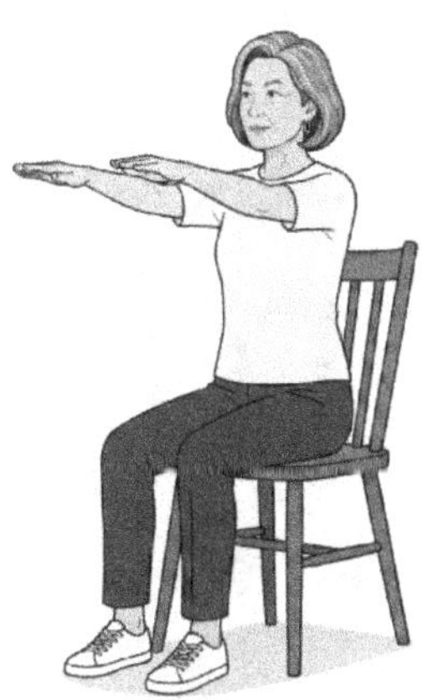

Form 2: Ward Off

Transfers body weight progressively to single-leg stance, building proprioceptive confidence while the arms establish the foundational guard position.

1. Shift weight slowly onto the left foot.

2. Raise the right arm to chest height, elbow bent, forearm crossing in front of the body, palm toward you. Lower the left arm to the hip. Right foot light, barely weighted. Left knee bent slightly deeper.

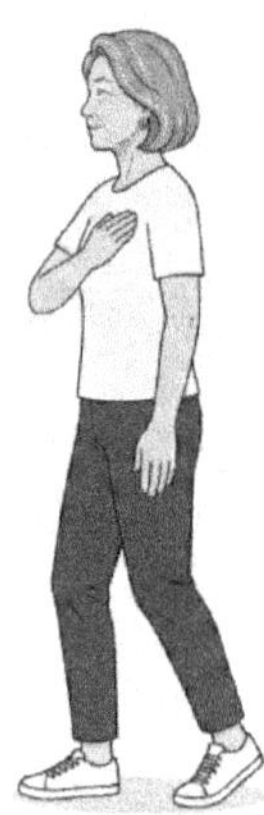

3. Hold for two breath cycles on the left foot.

4. Shift weight back to center. Lower the right arm.

5. Repeat on the right side: shift weight right, left arm rises, right arm lowers.

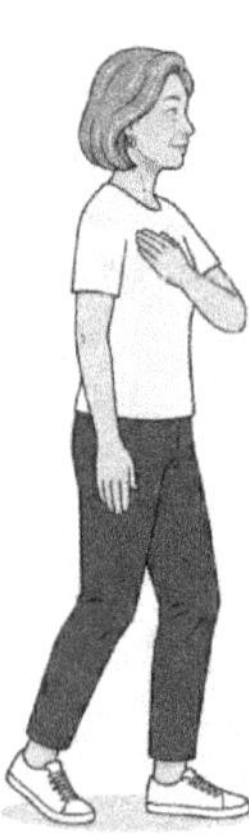

BREATHING: Inhale during the weight shift. Exhale as the position settles.

MIND NOTE: Name the three foot contact points (heel, ball, outer edge) during the hold to anchor attention.

JOINT NOTE: Single-leg loading drives synovial fluid through the knee and hip cartilage of the weighted leg.

BALANCE NOTE: Direct proprioceptive training for ankle and hip mechanoreceptors; allow the foot to find balance naturally without gripping with the toes.

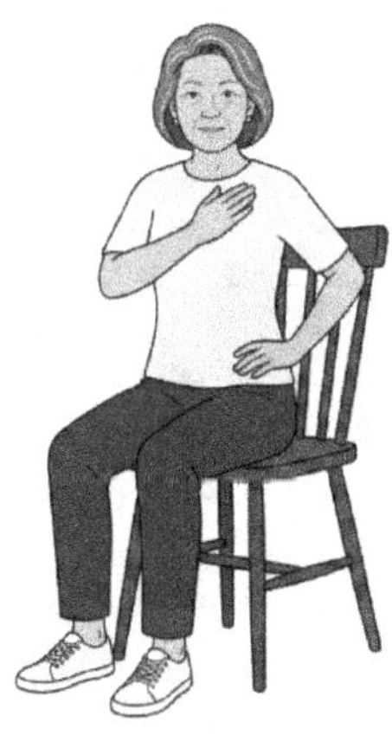

Form 3: Roll Back and Press

Trains sequential spinal and arm movement while lubricating the thoracic joints through continuous weight-shift coordination.

1. Take a small step forward with the right foot, shifting sixty percent of your weight forward with the right leg bent at the knee and bearing most of the body weight. Raise both arms forward to chest height, elbows bent, palms facing each other.

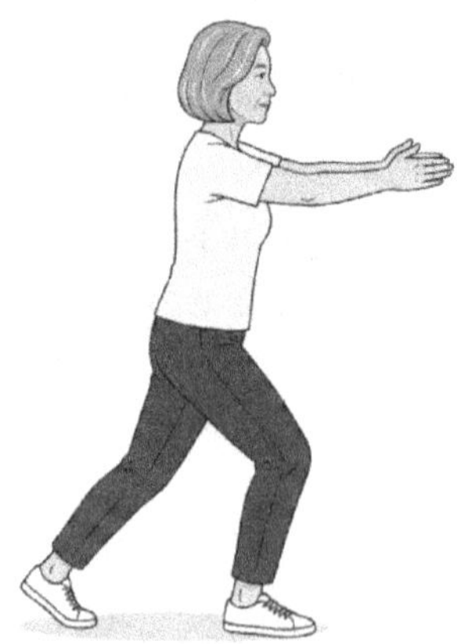

2. Inhale: draw both arms back (Roll Back) toward the chest, shifting weight to the back foot (left leg).

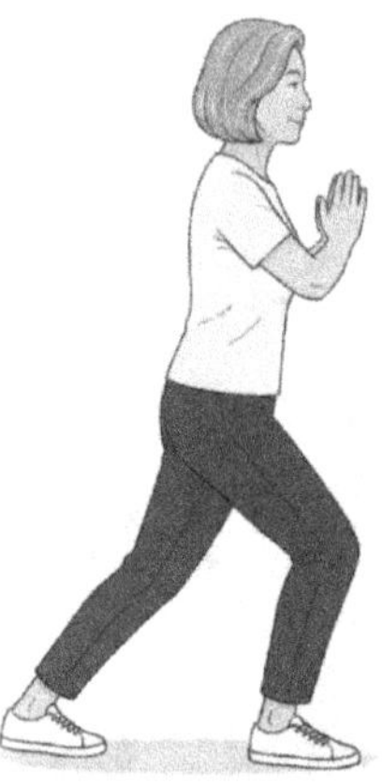

Exhale: press palms forward (Press), shifting weight to the front foot (right leg).

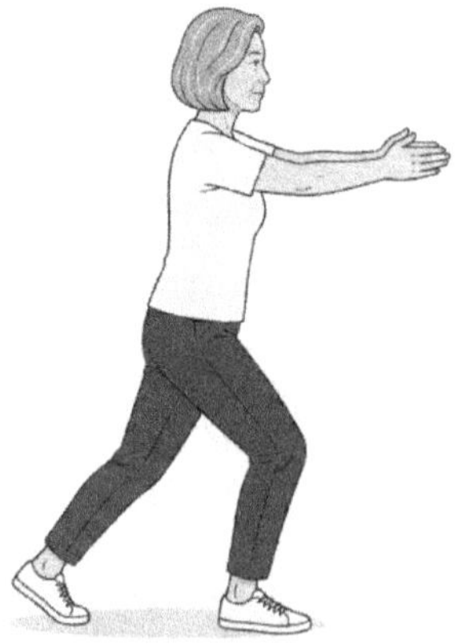

3. Complete four Roll Back-Press cycles. Step back. Repeat with left foot forward.

BREATHING: Inhale for Roll Back. Exhale for Press. The breath is the driver of each phase.

MIND NOTE: Track weight percentage under both feet simultaneously during each Roll Back and Press phase.

JOINT NOTE: Mobilizes the posterior shoulder capsule, the area most affected by chronic forward posture.

BALANCE NOTE: The forward-back weight shift replicates the proprioceptive mechanism of heel-to-toe rocking within a functional form.

WHAT THIS FORM DOES FOR YOU

Balance: The forward-back weight transfer between feet directly trains the same front-to-back stability your body needs to stop a stumble before it becomes a fall.

Joint Pain: The drawing-back motion opens the back of the shoulder capsule, which is one of the most commonly stiff areas in older adults who spend time at a desk or in a chair.

Mental Clarity: Tracking the weight shift under both feet simultaneously exercises the brain's spatial awareness, helping you feel more in control of your body in space.

SEATED MODIFICATION

Sit at the front of the chair. Draw the arms back on the inhale and press forward on the exhale. Thoracic and shoulder benefits are fully preserved.

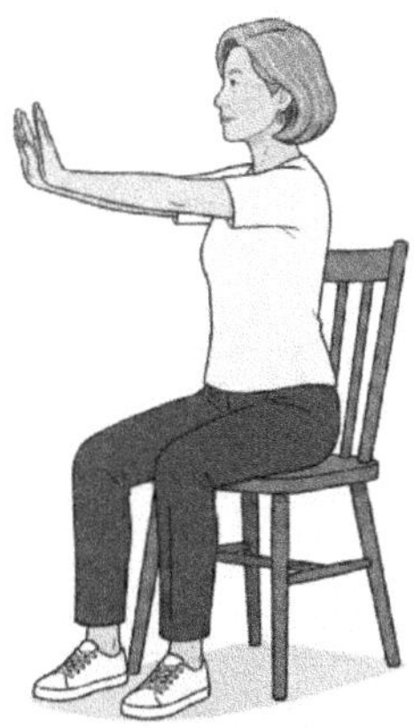

Form 4: White Crane Spreads Wings

Trains hip stability and shoulder range simultaneously; produces the most rapid proprioceptive feedback of the nine forms.

1. Step the right foot slightly back and to the right, leaving it light.

2. Shift all weight onto the left foot. The right toe tip touches the floor for reference only, bearing no weight.

3. Raise the left arm to chest height, palm angled forward and slightly upward, as if offering something. Drop the right arm to the right hip, palm facing back. The torso opens slightly to the right.

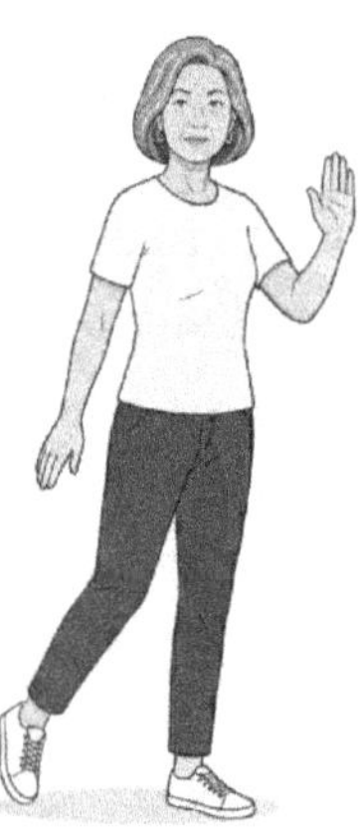

4. Hold for three breath cycles. Maintain the left foot balance. Keep the right toe contact light, as a reference point only.

5. Lower the left arm. Return the right foot to full weight. Shift to center.

6. Repeat on the right side: weight on right foot, right arm raises, left arm drops, left toe provides light contact.

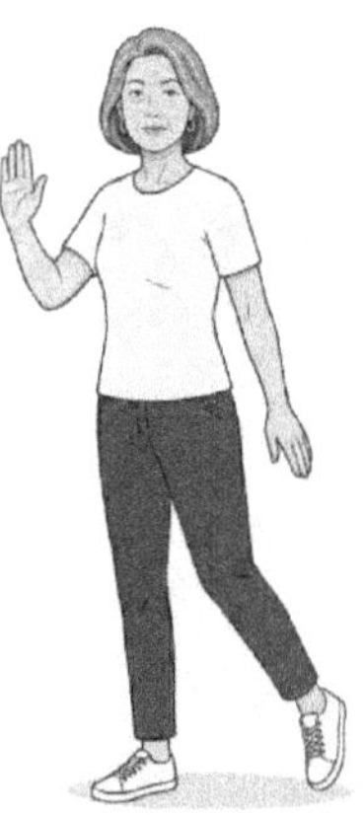

BREATHING: Breathe naturally through the hold. Do not restrict the breath to manage balance.

MIND NOTE: Alternate attention between standing foot contact and raised arm position as a working memory practice.

JOINT NOTE: Opens the shoulder joint through its superior arc, addressing compression from rounded shoulder posture.

BALANCE NOTE: Highest single-leg balance demand in early weeks; begin with fingertip chair contact and reduce support incrementally.

WHAT THIS FORM DOES FOR YOU

Balance: Holding full body weight on one foot for several breaths is direct, concentrated balance training that makes you steadier during everyday movements like dressing or stepping over obstacles.

Joint Pain: Raising one arm gently opens the top of the shoulder joint, which tends to compress and restrict from years of forward posture, reducing the overhead reach pain many seniors experience.

Mental Clarity: Alternating your focus between the standing foot and the raised arm is a deliberate mental exercise that builds the divided attention skill linked to sharper everyday thinking.

SEATED MODIFICATION

Sit at the front of the chair. Perform the arm positions. Shift lightly onto the corresponding sit-bone with each arm raise to preserve weight-shift coordination.

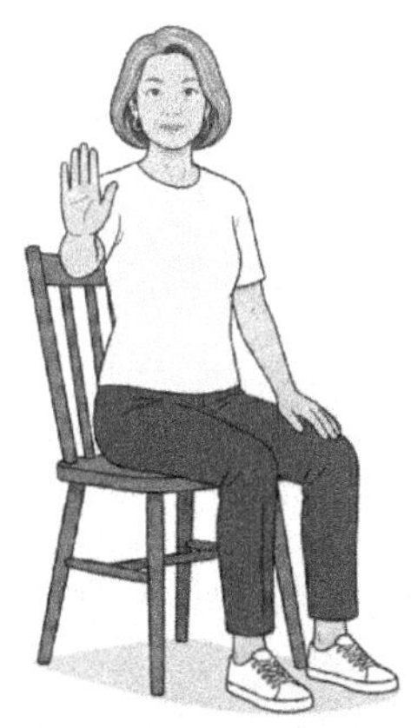

Form 5: Repulse the Monkey

Sequential weight transfer through alternating feet with an opposing arm push-pull; the highest coordination demand of the nine forms.

1. Step the left foot back one step, shifting weight fully onto it.

2. Extend the right hand forward at chest height, palm out. Draw the left hand to beside the left ear, palm forward.

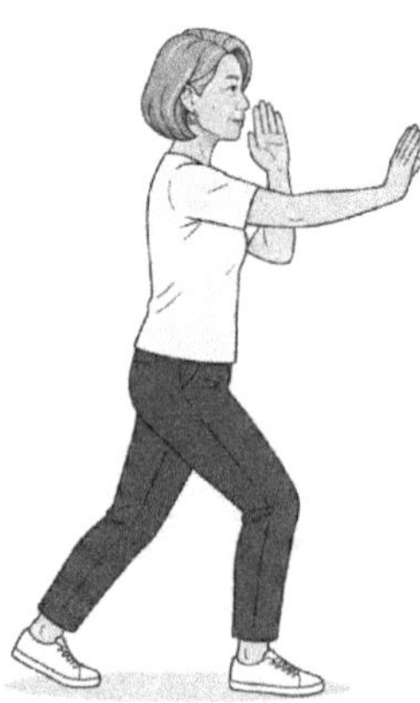

3. Step the right foot back. Shift weight onto the right foot.

4. The left hand extends forward while the right hand draws back to beside the right ear.

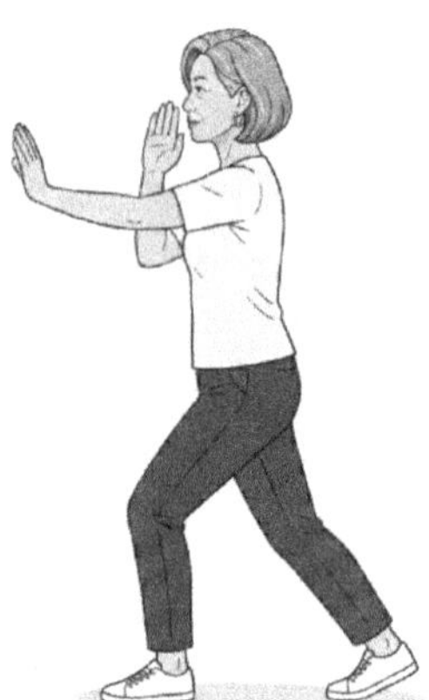

5. Continue alternating: step back, opposite arm extends, same-side arm draws to ear.

6. Complete four steps back each direction.

BREATHING: Inhale as the arm draws back to the ear. Exhale as the opposite arm extends forward.

MIND NOTE: The opposing simultaneous arm pattern is the program's highest bilateral coordination demand.

JOINT NOTE: Sequential hip compression and decompression on alternating sides, with posterior shoulder capsule work from the arm draw.

BALANCE NOTE: Each step back demands confident single-leg landing; backward stepping provides novel proprioceptive input beyond familiar forward patterns.

<hr>

WHAT THIS FORM DOES FOR YOU

Balance: Stepping backward is the movement your body uses to recover from a forward stumble. Practicing it deliberately makes that recovery faster and more reliable.

Joint Pain: The alternating step sequence compresses and releases the hip joints on both sides in turn, providing the movement stimulus the joint cartilage needs to stay healthy and less painful.

Mental Clarity: Coordinating opposite arms and legs simultaneously is one of the most challenging bilateral tasks in the program. It activates both sides of the brain at once, which research links to improved cognitive sharpness.

<hr>

SEATED MODIFICATION

Sit at the front of the chair. Alternate the arm push-pull pattern with each breath cycle. Cognitive and shoulder benefits fully preserved.

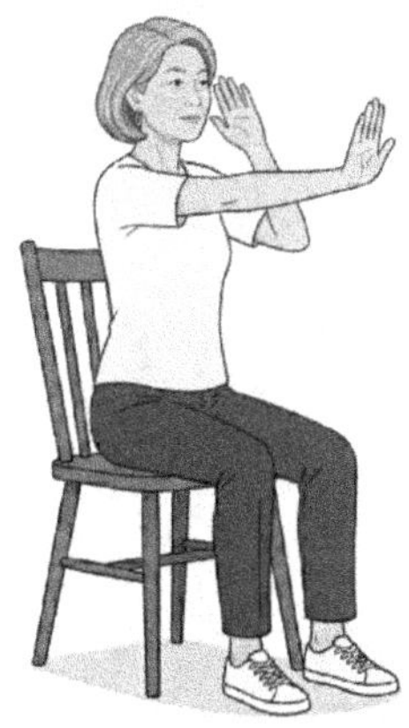

Form 6: Fair Lady Works the Shuttles

Introduces spinal rotation with synchronized arm elevation, addressing shoulder and hip rotation not provided by earlier forms.

1. Stand with feet shoulder-width apart, knees soft.

2. Turn the torso 45 degrees to the right. Allow the left foot to pivot to accommodate the turn.

3. Raise the left arm diagonally from the hip to above head, palm turning upward at the top. Lower the right arm to the right hip.

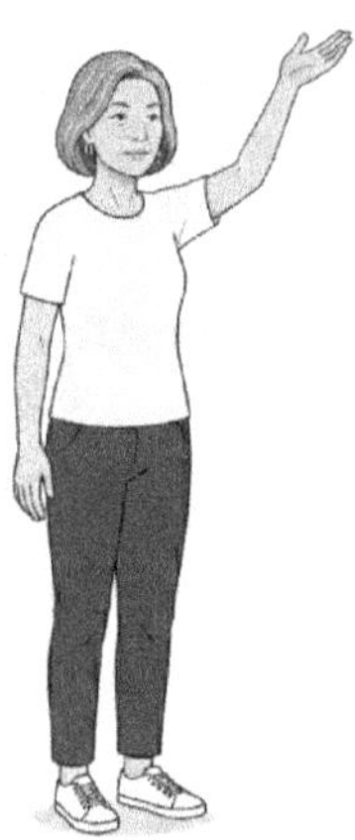

4. Hold for one breath cycle.

5. Lower the left arm and turn through center to 45 degrees left.

6. Raise the right arm above head height as described. Lower the left arm.

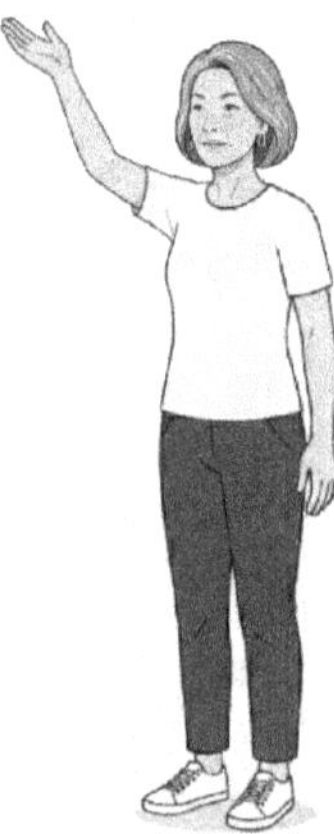

7. Hold for one breath cycle. Return through center.

BREATHING: Inhale as the arm rises. Exhale during the hold. Begin the turn on the next inhale.

MIND NOTE: Maintain foot-contact awareness during the turn; turning tends to reduce it and preserving it is the specific practice.

JOINT NOTE: Addresses the superior glenohumeral joint, most commonly restricted in older adults with rounded shoulder posture.

BALANCE NOTE: Turning while balancing requires vestibular recalibration as head orientation changes, providing direct vestibular training.

WHAT THIS DOES FOR YOU

Balance: Turning the body while keeping the feet grounded trains the vestibular system, which is the balance sensor in your inner ear that tells you which way is up when you pivot or turn.

Joint Pain: The diagonal arm raise addresses the top of the shoulder joint where compression from rounded posture is most common, helping to restore overhead reach and reduce shoulder aching.

Mental Clarity: Maintaining foot awareness during a turn is mentally demanding. It trains the attention-control skill that allows you to stay focused and safe when navigating busy or unpredictable environments.

SEATED MODIFICATION

Sit at the front of the chair. Turn the torso and raise the arm above head on each turn. Shoulder and thoracic rotation benefits are identical.

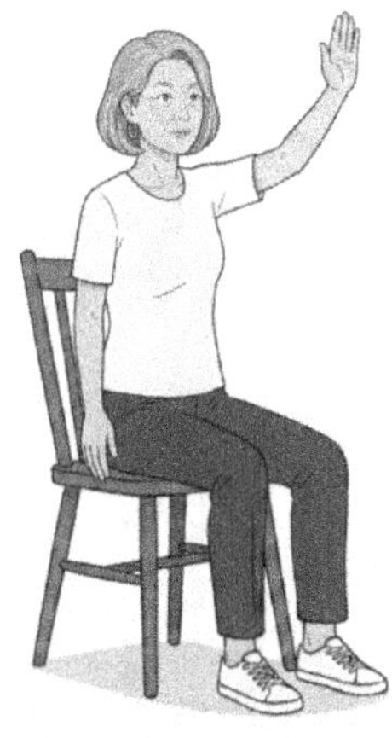

Form 7: Golden Rooster Stands on One Leg

Highest balance demand in the program; trains single-leg stability and hip flexion strength, with progress as the clearest proprioceptive measure.

1. Stand with feet flat.

2. Shift all weight slowly onto the right foot. Keep the right knee slightly bent, never locked.

3. Raise the left knee toward hip height, foot hanging naturally.

4. Raise the right arm forward to shoulder height simultaneously. The left arm hangs at the side.

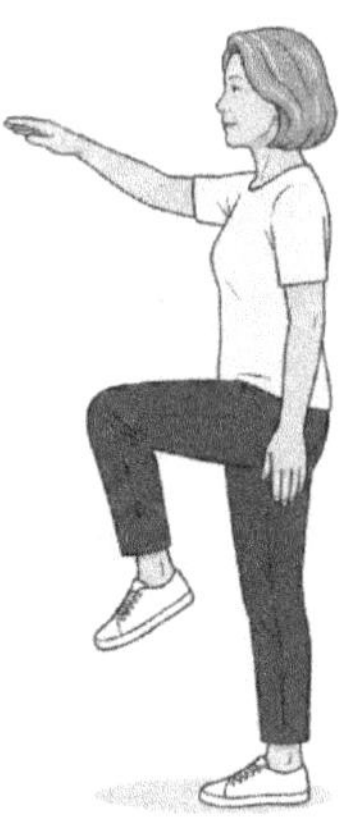

5. Hold for 3 to 10 seconds, building toward 30 seconds by Week 4.

6. Lower the left foot with control. Return to two-footed standing.

7. Repeat on the other side: weight on left foot, right knee raises, left arm raises.

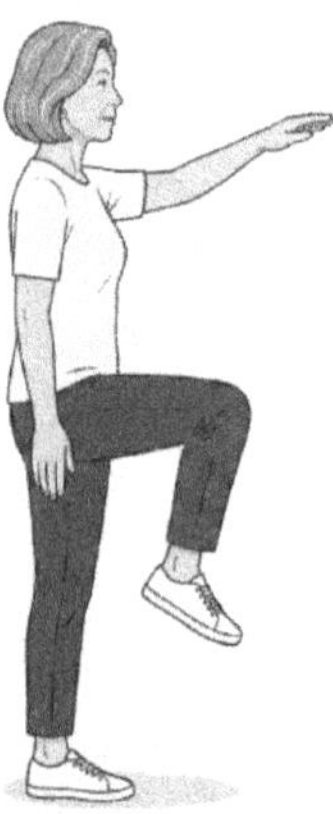

BREATHING: Breathe naturally throughout the hold. Breath-holding during balance challenges increases muscular tension and reduces balance quality.

MIND NOTE: Count the hold seconds silently; counting keeps prefrontal attention engaged and prevents balance-disrupting rumination.

JOINT NOTE: Hip flexion loading lubricates the flexion arc the hip rarely receives from sitting or lying, while the standing quadriceps strengthen under sustained single-leg load.

BALANCE NOTE: The most concentrated proprioceptive training in the program; ankle mechanoreceptor progress here is the clearest marker of proprioceptive improvement.

WHAT THIS DOES FOR YOU

Balance: Extended single-leg balance on one foot is the most direct balance training available. It strengthens the ankle, knee, and hip stabilizers that keep you upright when you hit an uneven surface.

Joint Pain: Raising the knee lubricates the hip joint through the range of motion that sitting and lying cannot provide, helping to ease the stiffness and aching in the hip flexors that many seniors experience in the morning.

Mental Clarity: Counting the hold seconds silently keeps the prefrontal cortex fully occupied, which is the same part of the brain used for planning, memory retrieval, and clear decision-making.

SEATED MODIFICATION

Sit at the front of the chair. Raise each knee toward the chest in turn, holding for five counts. Raise the opposite arm simultaneously.

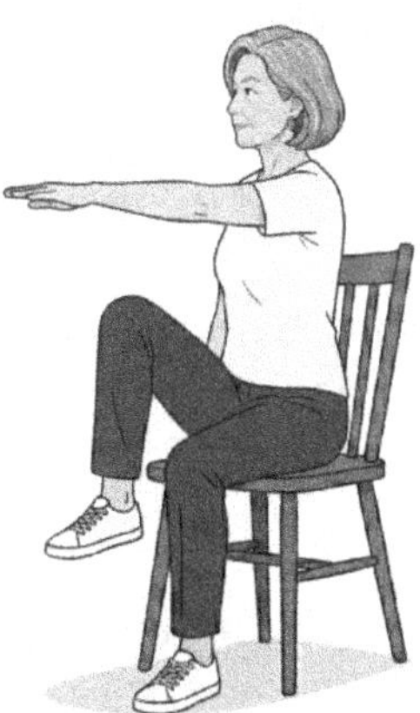

Form 8: Turn and Kick

Trains hip extension strength and the balance stability required for step-off-curb mechanics in real-world walking.

1. Stand with weight on both feet. Ensure clear space around you for the turn.

2. Shift weight onto the left foot. Extend the right leg gently backward a few inches, toes down. Float both arms forward for counterbalance.

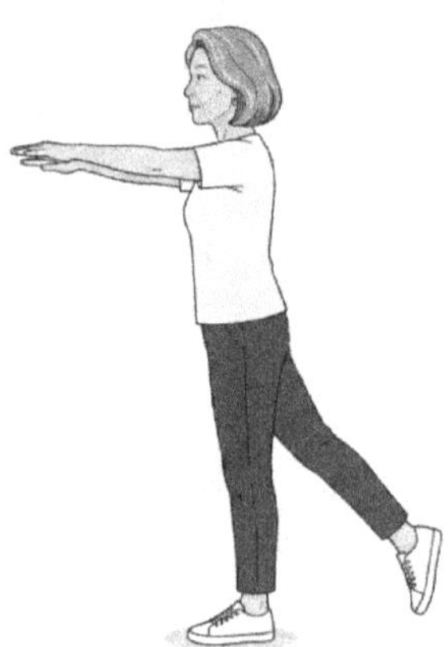

3. Hold two counts. Return the right foot.

4. Turn 90 degrees right, shifting weight to the right foot. Extend the left leg forward, foot flexed.

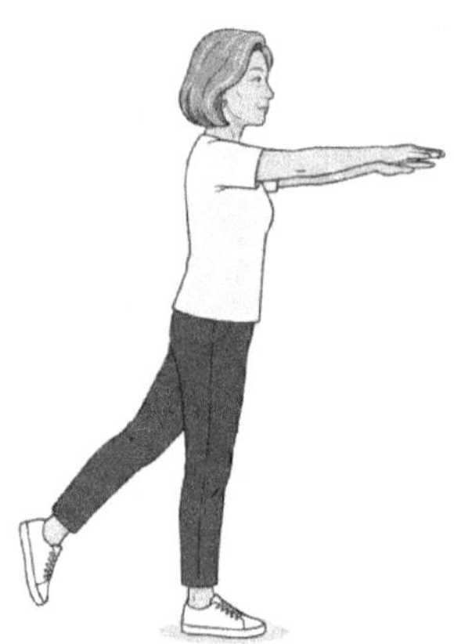

5. Hold two counts. Return the left foot. Turn back to center.

6. Repeat the sequence.

BREATHING: Inhale as each leg extends. Exhale during the hold.

MIND NOTE: Track where 'forward' is during and after the mid-form turn as a spatial reorientation exercise.

JOINT NOTE: Lubricates the posterior hip capsule, most compressed by prolonged sitting and most associated with morning hip stiffness.

BALANCE NOTE: The standing leg bears full body weight through a single joint chain, training the functional balance demand of stair-climbing and curb-stepping.

WHAT THIS DOES FOR YOU

Balance: The mid-form turn combined with a leg extension trains the coordination between your upper and lower body that is essential for navigating corners, doorways, and changing direction safely.

Joint Pain: Extending the leg behind and forward lubricates the back of the hip capsule, the area most compressed by prolonged sitting, and is directly associated with reducing the morning hip stiffness that many older adults experience.

Mental Clarity: Tracking your sense of direction during and after the turn challenges the brain's spatial orientation, a function that tends to decline with age and that this form specifically exercises.

SEATED MODIFICATION

Sit at the front of the chair. Extend each leg forward with foot flexed, holding for three counts.

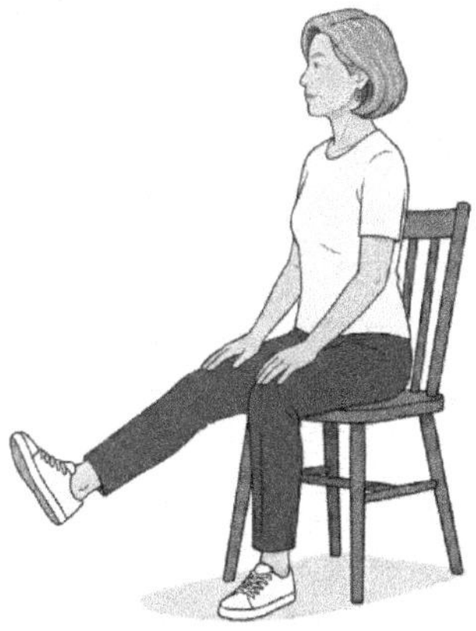

Form 9: Closing and Return

Mirrors Opening Form to signal session completion to the nervous system. Every session ends here, without exception.

1. Return to two-footed standing, weight even, knees soft. Pause for one breath cycle.

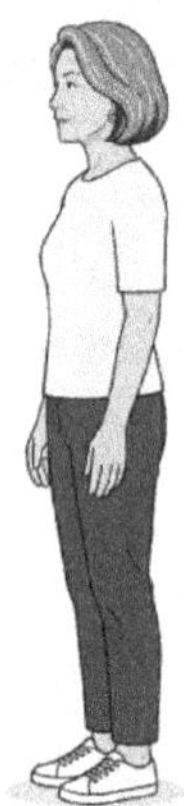

2. Raise both arms slowly to shoulder height, palms down. Slower than Opening Form.

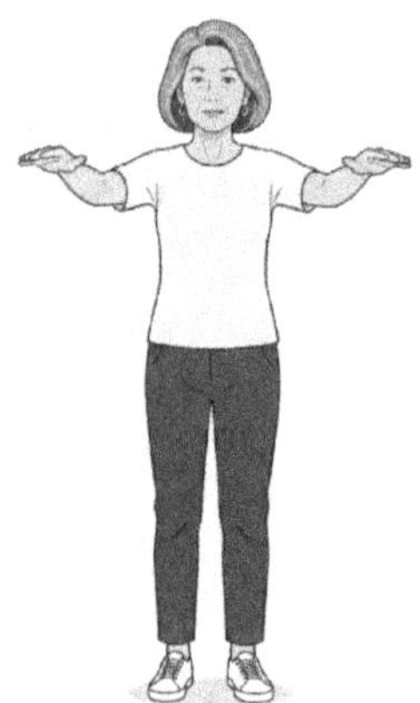

3. Hold at the top for one full inhale. Exhale and lower the arms slowly. Allow the exhale to extend fully.

4. Stand in stillness for three breath cycles. Notice body state and attention quality compared to session start.

5. When the three breath cycles are complete, the session is finished.

BREATHING: The exhale on the arm lowering should be at least twice as long as the inhale. This extended exhale is what completes the parasympathetic activation of the session.

MIND NOTE: Notice one specific body change from session start during the three closing breath cycles.

JOINT NOTE: The closing stillness allows reduced joint inflammation markers to settle at their new lower level before the day resumes.

BALANCE NOTE: The closing stillness is a balance assessment: compare stable standing quality now to the start of Opening Form.

WHAT THIS DOES FOR YOU

Balance: The slow stillness of the closing posture allows your balance system to register a stable endpoint, reinforcing the proprioceptive reference point your body uses for everyday upright standing.

Joint Pain: The extended exhale during the close signals the nervous system to reduce muscle tension and lower inflammation markers in the joints, compounding the physical benefits of the entire session.

Mental Clarity: The deliberate closing breath practice activates the parasympathetic nervous system, which calms mental chatter, reduces cortisol, and leaves your mind clearer and more focused for the rest of the day.

SEATED MODIFICATION

Sit at the front of the chair. Perform the arm rise and lower. Three closing breath cycles identical seated.

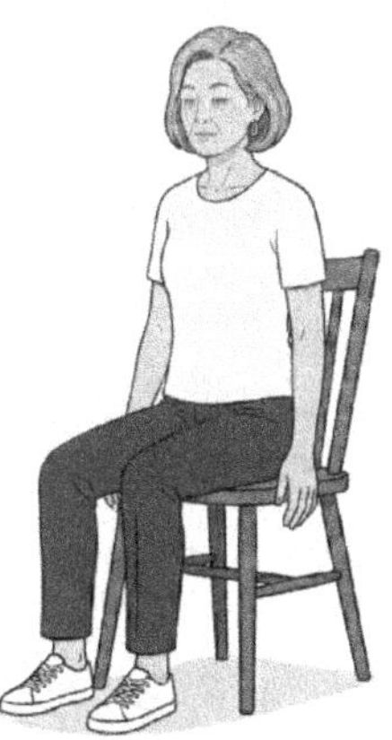

Breath Timing for Every Movement

One rule applies across all nine forms: the exhale is always longer than the inhale. If breath and movement lose coordination, restore the breath before restoring the form position. Maintained breath with imprecise positions is more beneficial than precise positions with held breath. Breath coordination resolves naturally by Week Two.

Common Mistakes and How to Spot Them

Six common errors. Each has a WHY IT MATTERS note and a three-step correction with images.

Mistake 1: Locked Knees

Standing with both knees fully straight throughout the session removes the shock-absorbing function of the knee joint and places excessive load on the joint surfaces. It also reduces the proprioceptive input from the knee mechanoreceptors, which require slight flexion to operate optimally.

WHY IT MATTERS: Locked knees during weight-shifting increase cartilage impingement risk and reduce proprioceptive input from the knee mechanoreceptors.

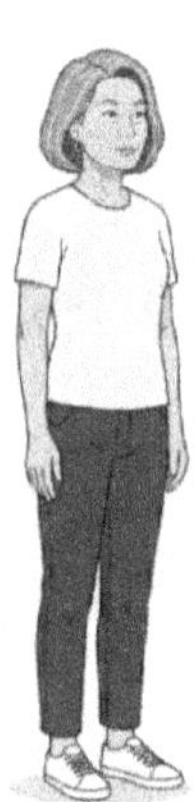

CORRECTION:

1. Stand with feet shoulder-width apart.

2. Release the knees approximately ten degrees from straight.

3. Hold: the feeling is as if you began to sit down and stopped early.

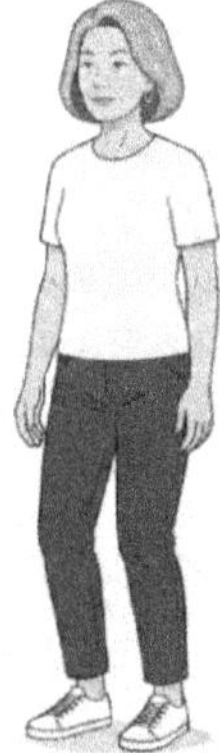

Mistake 2: Raised Shoulders

Lifting the shoulders toward the ears during the forms compresses the cervical spine, restricts shoulder mobility, and signals threat to the nervous system rather than safety.

WHY IT MATTERS: Chronic shoulder elevation during practice prevents the shoulder joint lubrication the forms are designed to provide and sustains the cortisol-associated tension response.

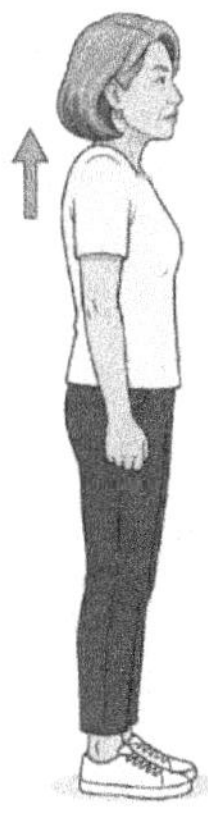

CORRECTION:

1. Inhale at the start of each form.

2. Exhale and actively drop the shoulders away from the ears.

3. Re-check shoulder position at the midpoint of each form.

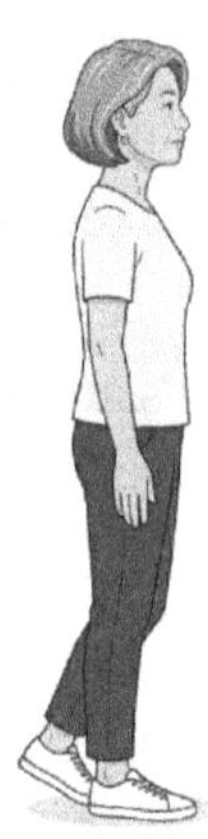

Mistake 3: Gaze Directed at the Feet

Looking down at the feet reduces the visual field needed for environmental awareness and places the cervical spine in sustained flexion.

WHY IT MATTERS: Forward gaze is essential for vestibular balance function. Downward gaze shifts the center of mass forward, increasing fall risk.

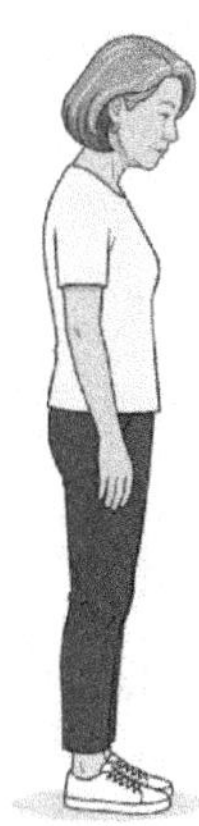

CORRECTION:

1. Choose a wall point at eye level before each session.

2. Return the gaze to this point at the start of each new form.

3. In turning forms (Fair Lady, Turn and Kick), follow the turn then return to eye-level forward gaze.

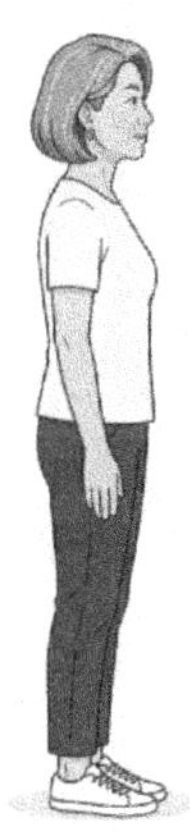

WHY FIXING THIS HELPS YOU

Balance: Your balance system uses three inputs: the feet, the inner ear, and the eyes. When the eyes are looking down, they stop contributing useful information and the balance system becomes less reliable. Eyes forward restores the full three-input system.

Joint Pain: Looking down pulls the head forward and compresses the back of the neck. Over a ten-minute session, this adds up to significant strain. A level gaze keeps the spine in its natural, load-bearing alignment.

Mistake 4: Holding the Breath

Breath-holding during balance-demanding holds is an automatic stress response, extremely common in the first week when balance challenges activate mild threat responses.

WHY IT MATTERS: Held breath activates the sympathetic nervous system, undoing the cortisol-reduction effect that is one of the primary benefits of the practice.

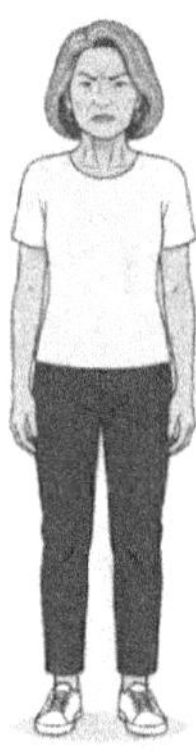
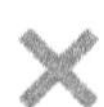

CORRECTION:

1. If you notice breath-holding, exhale completely before resuming.
2. In Golden Rooster, speak one word aloud during the hold: speaking is impossible while holding the breath.
3. Reduce balance demand with chair support until breath maintains naturally through the hold.

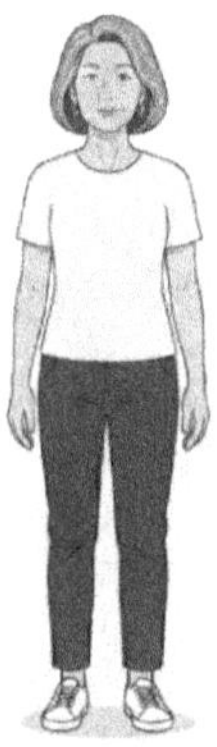

Mistake 5: Weight Not Fully Transferred

Partial weight transfer in single-weight forms (Ward Off, White Crane, Golden Rooster) reduces the proprioceptive training effect and makes the forms easier than intended.

WHY IT MATTERS: Incomplete weight transfer reduces the proprioceptive training signal proportionally. The mechanoreceptors need full single-leg loading to be effectively trained.

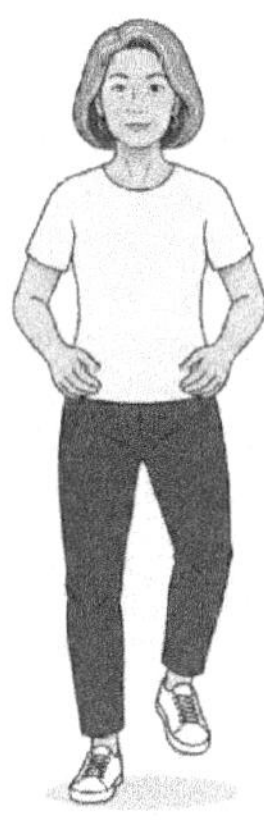
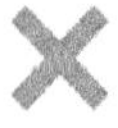

CORRECTION:

1. Identify the standing foot before the form begins.

2. Press the standing sole into the floor and shift until the other foot is genuinely light.

3. Test by lifting the light foot slightly: significant wobble means the transfer was incomplete.

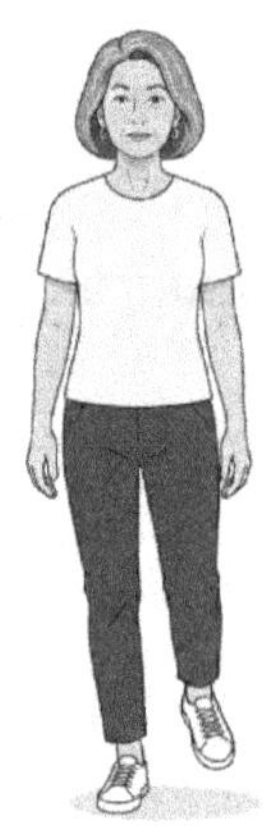

Mistake 6: Arms and Legs Moving Out of Coordination

In coordination-intensive forms (Repulse the Monkey, Turn and Kick), arms and legs frequently drift out of the simultaneous pattern, with one completing before the other begins.

WHY IT MATTERS: Asynchronous movement reduces the bilateral coordination demand and therefore the working memory and cognitive benefit of the form.

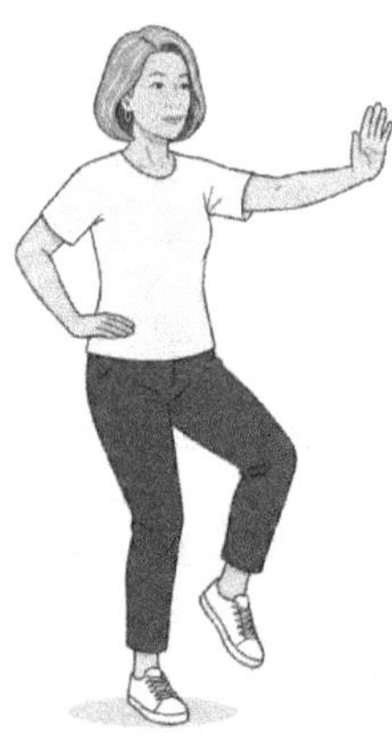

CORRECTION:

1. Slow down. Coordination errors almost always indicate moving faster than the nervous system can manage.

2. Practice arm and foot movements separately, then combine at half speed.

3. Coordination is correct when both movements arrive at their positions simultaneously.

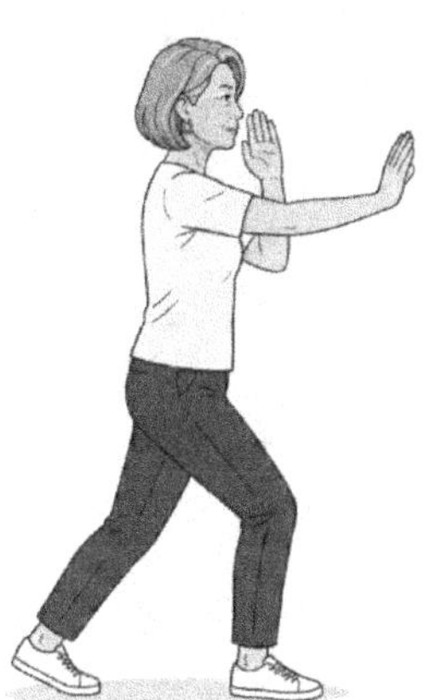

> **WHY FIXING THIS HELPS YOU**
>
> **Balance:** Coordinated arm and leg movement is what makes the body move as a unified whole rather than as separate parts. When they are synchronised, the arms act as counterweights that stabilise the entire walking and standing pattern.
>
> **Joint Pain:** Asynchronous movement causes uneven torque through the spine and hip joints as each side of the body tries to compensate for the timing gap. Synchronised movement distributes forces evenly, reducing strain on the joints.
>
> **Mental Clarity:** Getting both limbs to arrive at their positions at exactly the same time is a genuine bilateral brain exercise. Slowing down and achieving that synchronisation is one of the most cognitively rewarding moments in the practice.

Balance Builders

These four exercises appear from Week Three onward, performed at the end of the session before Closing and Return. Each targets a specific proprioceptive mechanism. Step count restarts at 1 for each exercise.

Balance Builder 1: Tandem Stand

Trains narrow-base balance stability for confined-space navigation.

1. Stand beside the chair with one hand available for support.

2. Place the right foot heel-to-toe in front of the left.

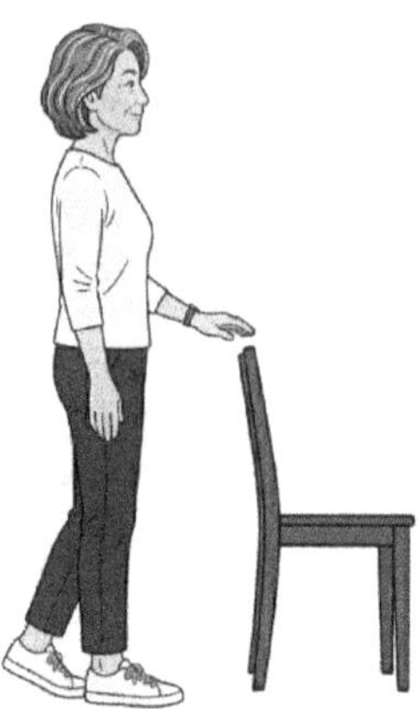

3. Release the chair. Hold for 10 to 30 seconds.

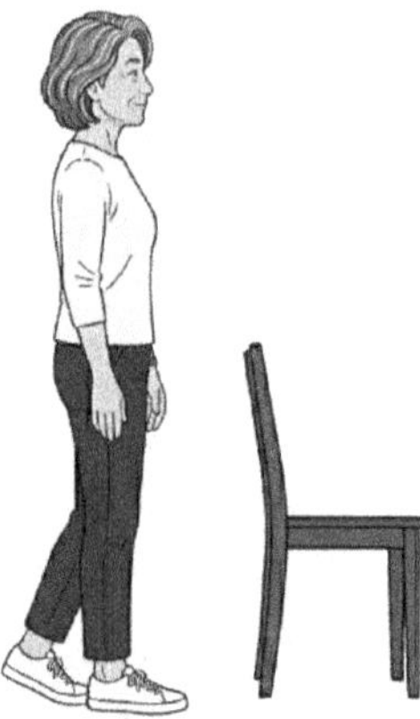

4. If balance fails, touch the chair. Switch feet and hold.

BALANCE NOTE: The narrow base forces ankle mechanoreceptors to manage all lateral perturbations, the most specific proprioceptive drill for step-to-step stability.

WHAT THIS DOES FOR YOU

Balance: Standing heel-to-toe on a narrow line is the closest thing to a real walking step that a standing exercise can provide. Training this position builds the ankle stability you use for every step you take on uneven ground, in a crowd, or on a sloped surface.

Joint Pain: Holding the tandem position gently loads the ankle and knee in their natural alignment without any impact, promoting the joint fluid circulation that reduces stiffness without adding strain.

Balance Builder 2: Heel Raise with Eyes Closed

Removes visual balance input to train complete reliance on proprioception and vestibular input under reduced-visibility conditions.

1. Stand behind the chair, hands lightly on the back. Rise onto the balls of both feet.

2. Hold for five counts, then lower heels slowly.

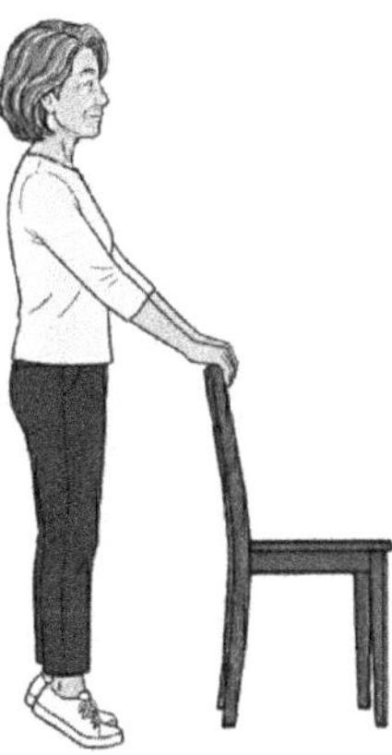

3. Next repetition: close the eyes before rising. Open them before lowering.

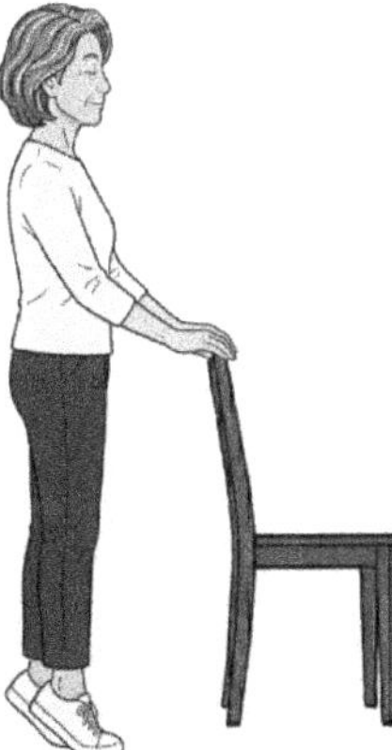

4. Complete 5 repetitions with eyes open, 5 with eyes closed.

BALANCE NOTE: Eyes-closed heel raise completely isolates proprioceptive and vestibular inputs, revealing how much visual compensation was masking proprioceptive deficit.

WHAT THIS DOES FOR YOU

Balance: Closing your eyes removes the visual safety net that most people rely on more than they realise. When the eyes are closed, the feet and ankles must do the entire job of managing balance. This is exactly the situation you face in a dark hallway or dimly lit space, and this exercise trains you for it directly.

Joint Pain: Rising onto the balls of the feet repeatedly pumps blood and synovial fluid through the ankle joint and stretches the Achilles tendon, which is one of the most common sources of morning stiffness in older adults.

Mental Clarity: The heightened concentration required when your eyes are closed sharpens interoceptive awareness, the ability to sense your own body from the inside, which is the same quality that makes the Tai Chi forms more effective with each week of practice.

Balance Builder 3: Lateral Weight Shift

Trains hip stabilizers through slow side-to-side weight transfer to prevent hip-drop during single-leg walking phases.

1. Stand with feet slightly wider than shoulder-width.

2. Shift weight slowly right over five counts. Allow the right knee to deepen. Left leg extended but foot flat. Keep hips level.

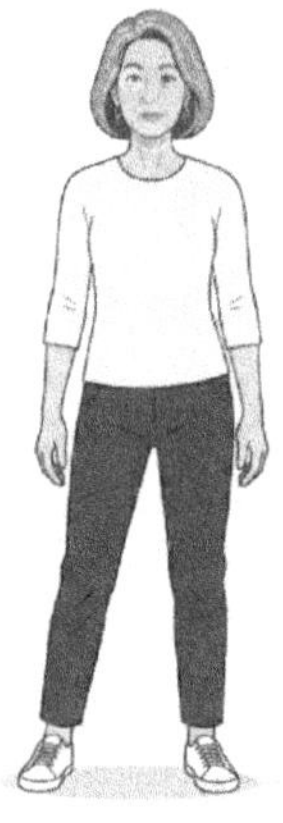 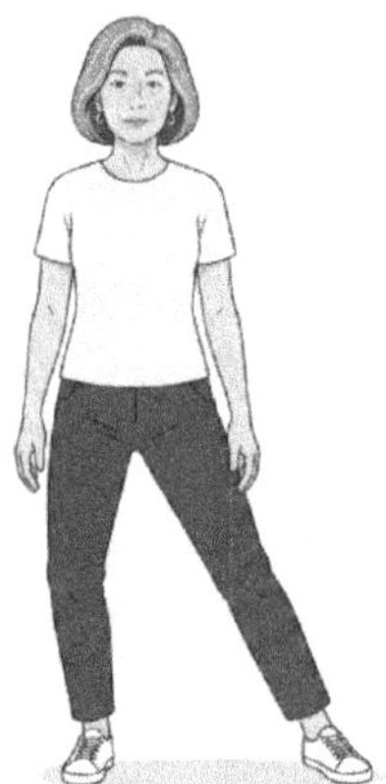

3. Hold at the right for two counts.

4. Shift back through center and continue left over five counts.

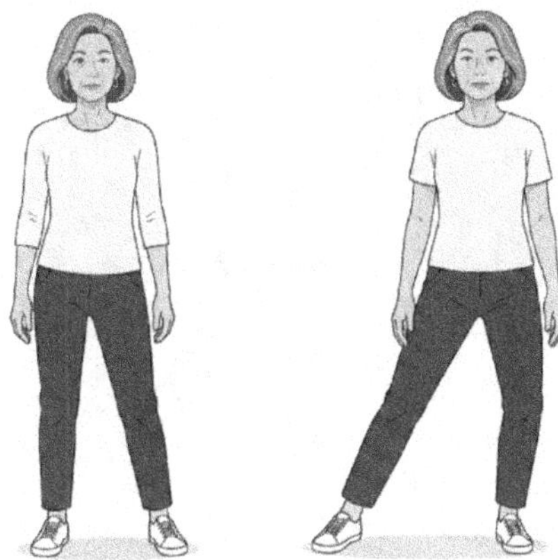

5. Hold left for two counts. Return to center.

6. Complete 6 full cycles.

BALANCE NOTE: Slow speed prevents momentum, requiring every increment of the shift to be actively managed by the hip stabilizers, providing direct gluteus medius training.

> **WHAT THIS DOES FOR YOU**
>
> **Balance:** Most falls happen sideways, not forward. The muscles on the outside of the hip (the gluteus medius) are responsible for preventing a sideways drop when one foot leaves the ground. This exercise targets those muscles directly, in the slow deliberate way that builds reliable real-world stability.
>
> **Joint Pain:** The slow lateral shift compresses and releases the hip joints in the side-to-side plane that ordinary forward walking does not address. This helps to lubricate the areas of hip cartilage that are most often missed by other exercises.
>
> **Mental Clarity:** Maintaining a level pelvis while the weight moves sideways requires sustained attention that is different in quality from forward movement. Focusing on keeping the hips level gives the mind a precise, achievable task that builds the concentration habits the forms reward.

Balance Builder 4: Single-Leg Reach

Advances single-leg balance with a reaching challenge that shifts the center of mass, replicating daily-life reaching demands.

1. Shift weight onto the right foot, left foot slightly lifted.

2. Extend the right arm forward and slightly downward, allowing the torso to hinge forward slightly. Left leg slightly behind for stability

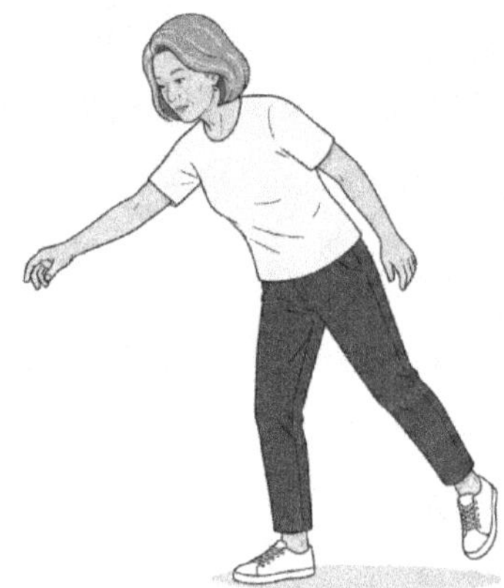

3. Hold for three counts. Return upright. Complete 3 reaches each side, then switch standing foot.

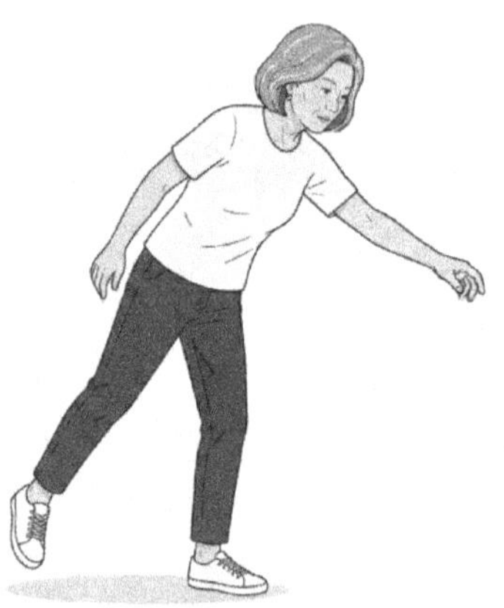

BALANCE NOTE: The forward reach displaces the center of mass outside the base, requiring hip stabilizers and ankle dorsiflexors to produce a corrective moment, replicating the balance demand of every daily-life reach.

WHAT THIS DOES FOR YOU

Balance: Reaching forward while standing on one foot mimics dozens of real-life moments: picking something up from a low surface, reaching across a table, opening a low cupboard. Training this movement in a controlled setting makes all those moments steadier and safer.

Joint Pain: The hip of the standing leg works through an extended range during the forward lean, providing the type of hip extension loading that is most effective at reducing the deep hip stiffness that comes from sitting for long periods.

Mental Clarity: The reach adds a spatial planning element to the balance challenge. The brain must simultaneously calculate the forward movement and manage the standing balance, which is a more demanding and more rewarding mental exercise than either task alone.

A Small Request

If working through this book has done something useful for you even one small thing that shifted, it would mean a great deal to hear about it. Would you be willing to leave a short, honest review on Amazon?

As an independent author, books like this one find their readers through honest reviews not advertising, not algorithms, just one person telling another that something helped them. If the past 4 chapters read so far produced any change you would want someone else to know about, a short review on Amazon is the most direct way to pass that along.

Two minutes. One or two sentences. That is genuinely all it takes, and it matters more than most people realize.

You can leave your review on Amazon by searching the title ***Standing Tai Chi for Seniors Over 60 by Liuhe Chen*** on Amazon. It takes two minutes, and it matters more than you know.

Chapter 5

The 28-Day Program

This is the operational program. Read the week overview before the first session of each new week. Read the coaching note before each session. It changes what follows.

The nine forms are introduced progressively. Each week contains two scheduled rest days placed on the days where recovery is most beneficial for older bodies. Rest days are marked clearly. Do not replace a scheduled rest day with a practice session. The adaptation this program produces happens during rest, not during effort alone.

Every practice day uses the same format: a Session At a Glance box, a coaching note from Liuhe Ming, and a NOTICE TODAY prompt. The NOTICE TODAY prompt changes each day and each week. It is not decorative. Every practice day also includes a low-energy option of no more than five minutes for days when energy or joint comfort is limited. Use it without guilt.

Week 1 – Grounded and Still

Three forms this week: Opening Form, Ward Off, and Closing and Return. Sessions are ten minutes. The week is about establishing the foundational standing posture and breath pattern before adding movement complexity. The forms are simple. The quality of attention to them is not.

Most people find the first two sessions cognitively tiring in proportion to their brief physical duration. This is the prefrontal cortex building new motor programs, a genuinely effortful neural process. By Day 3 the cognitive load reduces as the forms begin to feel familiar. By Day 5 the breath coordination becomes less effortful to maintain.

What You Might Feel This Week
- A mild cognitive tiredness after the early sessions. This is the brain working, not the practice being too hard.

• The Ward Off weight shift may feel uncertain on the standing foot. This is the proprioceptive system reporting accurately. It will improve.

• A brief settling sensation in the joints during the Closing and Return stillness. This is the synovial circulation effect of the forms beginning to operate.

Your Win This Week: Complete every practice session, regardless of how the forms feel. Completion is the only standard this week.

Day 1 – Ground and Breathe

SESSION AT A GLANCE
10 minutes | Forms: Opening Form, Ward Off (3 each side), Closing and Return | Low-energy option: Opening Form and breath only, 3 minutes

Liuhe's Note:
Before anything else, do the Day One Self-Assessment from Chapter Three if you have not already. Record the three numbers. Then stand in your practice space and take one breath before beginning Opening Form. The breath before the form begins the transition from ordinary morning awareness into the practice. Do not skip it.

NOTICE TODAY:
During Ward Off, notice which foot feels more stable as the standing foot. Most people have a dominant balance side. Knowing yours from Day 1 is useful information.

Day 2 – Finding the Weight

SESSION AT A GLANCE
10 minutes | Forms: Opening Form, Ward Off, Closing and Return | Focus: complete weight transfer in Ward Off | Low-energy option: Opening Form and Ward Off one side only, 4 minutes

Liuhe's Note:
The key question today is whether the weight is transferring fully onto the standing foot in Ward Off, or whether the other foot is still carrying some weight as a safety measure. Both are acceptable at this stage. Notice which it is. Full transfer is the target. It will come.

NOTICE TODAY:

Place one hand lightly on the chair during Ward Off if needed. Notice whether the hand is actually needed or simply reassuring. There is a difference, and knowing the difference tells you something about your balance confidence.

Day 3 – The Breath Coordination

SESSION AT A GLANCE
10 minutes | Forms: Opening Form, Ward Off, Closing and Return | Focus: breath timing through all three forms | Low-energy option: Opening Form and Closing and Return, 3 minutes

Liuhe's Note:
Today's attention is on the breath. Inhale as the arms rise in Opening Form. Exhale as they lower. Inhale during the Ward Off weight shift. Exhale as the position settles. If the breath and the movement lose coordination at any point, stop, exhale completely, and continue. The breath is always the priority.

NOTICE TODAY:
Notice whether holding the Ward Off position is easier or harder on the third session compared to Day 1. Any reduction in effort is the nervous system building the motor program.

Day 4 – Rest

REST DAY
No formal practice session today. Rest is part of the program.

Liuhe's Note:
Day 4 is a scheduled rest day. The neural consolidation of what the first three sessions built happens now, during rest, not during practice. Take a short walk or do gentle stretching if the body wants movement. Do not do the standing forms today.

Day 5 – Back to Standing

SESSION AT A GLANCE
10 minutes | Forms: Opening Form, Ward Off, Closing and Return | Focus: comparing today to Day 3 | Low-energy option: Opening Form only with three breath cycles, 3 minutes

Liuhe's Note:

Most people find the first session after a rest day noticeably more settled than the one before it. The forms feel slightly more familiar. The weight transfer in Ward Off is slightly more confident. Pay attention to this. The improvement happened during the rest day, not during today's session.

NOTICE TODAY:
Balance, joints, or breath: which of the three feels most different today compared to Day 1? Name one specific thing.

Day 6 – Stillness Practice

SESSION AT A GLANCE
10 minutes | Forms: Opening Form, Ward Off (extended holds), Closing and Return | Focus: extending the Ward Off hold to 5 breath cycles | Low-energy option: Opening Form and Closing and Return only, 5 minutes

Liuhe's Note:
Today extend the Ward Off hold to five full breath cycles on each side. Five cycles is approximately forty seconds. If the balance is not yet stable for forty seconds, hold for as many cycles as possible, rest for one breath, and continue. Building the hold duration is the proprioceptive training target this week.

NOTICE TODAY:
During the extended Ward Off hold, is the quality of attention sustained through all five cycles, or does the mind wander after two or three? Attention endurance is as much a practice outcome as balance endurance.

Day 7 – Rest

REST DAY
No formal practice session today. Rest is part of the program.

Liuhe's Note:
Week One ends with a rest day. The nervous system and joints benefit most from recovery before the new demands of Week Two arrive. Take a short walk or sit quietly. Do not practice the standing forms today.

Learning to Stand Before You Move

Week One establishes a foundation that every subsequent week depends on: the quality of standing itself. Most people arrive at this practice with decades of habitual standing posture, much of which involves shifted weight, locked joints, and held tension. The three forms of Week One ask for something specific and different: weight evenly distributed, joints mobile, breath continuing, attention present. Getting these things established before the movement complexity of Week Two is the function of this week. It is not a beginner's compromise. It is the practice.

Managing Stiffness in the First Week

Joint stiffness in the first week of a new movement practice is not a sign that the practice is wrong for the body. It is the joints encountering movement demands that daily life has not been providing. The stiffness typically peaks on the second or third day and begins to ease from Day 4 or 5 onward. Reducing the depth of the knee bend in Ward Off and reducing the duration of the holds manages the stiffness without abandoning the practice. Stopping the practice in response to the stiffness removes the mechanism that resolves the stiffness.

Week 2 – Open the Joints

This week adds White Crane Spreads Wings and Repulse the Monkey to the sequence. Sessions extend to twelve minutes. The two new forms introduce single-leg balance demands beyond Ward Off and a stepping coordination pattern that requires simultaneous bilateral arm and leg management.

The week theme of opening the joints refers specifically to the synovial fluid distribution effect that the new forms provide to the hip, shoulder, and thoracic joints. By the end of this week, most people notice a difference in the morning stiffness pattern compared to Week One. The forms are producing cumulative joint lubrication that is beginning to outlast the sessions.

What You Might Feel This Week

- The stepping pattern of Repulse the Monkey is the most coordination-demanding sequence introduced so far. Expect it to feel rough for the first two sessions. It settles.
- Joint warmth during and after the session, particularly in the hips and shoulders. This is the increased synovial fluid circulation, not inflammation.

- The Ward Off single-leg hold may already feel more stable than it did on Day 1. This is the beginning of the proprioceptive improvement that Week Three will deepen.

Your Win This Week: Perform Repulse the Monkey with the arm and leg movements arriving at their positions simultaneously on at least one repetition.

Day 8 – Two New Forms

SESSION AT A GLANCE
12 minutes | Forms: Opening Form, Ward Off, White Crane, Repulse the Monkey, Closing and Return | Low-energy option: Opening Form, Ward Off, Closing and Return only, 5 mins

Liuhe's Note:
Two new forms today. Learn White Crane first: read the form description again, then practice it three times before adding Repulse the Monkey. Do not attempt to run the full sequence on Day 8. The session is for learning, not flowing.

NOTICE TODAY:
During White Crane, which hip feels more stable as the standing hip? Note it. The weaker hip stabilizer is the one that benefits most from this form.

Day 9 – The Stepping Pattern

SESSION AT A GLANCE
12 minutes | All five forms | Focus: Repulse the Monkey arm and foot timing | Low-energy option: Opening Form, White Crane, Closing and Return, 5 minutes

Liuhe's Note:
The most common error in Repulse the Monkey is the arms and feet arriving at their positions at different times. Slow the form to half speed and focus on a single step: as the foot reaches its landing position, the opposite arm reaches its extended position simultaneously. If they are not simultaneous, slow down further.

NOTICE TODAY:
Notice which direction of stepping in Repulse the Monkey feels more natural. Most people have a directional preference that reflects an asymmetry in the hip stabilizers.

Day 10 – Rest

<table><tr><td>

REST DAY
No formal practice session today. Rest is part of the program.

</td></tr><tr><td>

Liuhe's Note:
This rest day arrives after two sessions with the new forms. White Crane and Repulse the Monkey introduce significant hip and shoulder demands. Let the joints consolidate today. Tomorrow the sequence will feel clearer.

</td></tr></table>

Day 11 – Hip Opening

<table><tr><td>

SESSION AT A GLANCE
12 minutes | All five forms | Focus: the hip joint experience in White Crane and Repulse | Low-energy option: Opening Form, White Crane, Closing and Return, 5 minutes

</td></tr><tr><td>

Liuhe's Note:
Today bring attention specifically to the hip of the standing leg during White Crane, and then to the alternating hip loading during Repulse the Monkey. Both forms are doing significant synovial work in the hip joints. Notice whether the hip feels different at the end of the session from the beginning.

</td></tr><tr><td>

NOTICE TODAY:
Can you feel the difference in the hip joint between the first repetition of White Crane and the third? The third should feel more mobile. That is the synovial fluid distributing.

</td></tr></table>

Day 12 – Sequence Flow

<table><tr><td>

SESSION AT A GLANCE
12 minutes | All five forms in continuous sequence | Focus: transitions between forms | Low-energy option: Opening Form, Ward Off, White Crane, Closing and Return, 5 minutes

</td></tr><tr><td>

Liuhe's Note:
Today run all five forms in continuous sequence without stopping between them. The transition from one form to the next is part of the practice. Use the Closing and Return stillness at the end to notice the state of the joints after a continuous sequence.

</td></tr><tr><td>

NOTICE TODAY:
Which transition between forms feels least smooth? That is tomorrow's specific focus.

</td></tr></table>

Day 13 – Rest

> **REST DAY**
> No formal practice session today. Rest is part of the program.

> **Liuhe's Note:**
> The second rest day of Week Two comes before the Day 14 joint comfort check. Measuring from a recovered state produces a more honest result than measuring through fatigue. Rest fully today.

Day 14 – Joint Comfort Check

> **SESSION AT A GLANCE**
> 12 minutes | All five forms | Focus: honest comparison to the Chapter Three baseline | Low-energy option: Opening Form, White Crane, Closing and Return, 5 minutes

> **Liuhe's Note:**
> Two weeks complete. Before the session, retrieve your Day One stiffness rating from Chapter Three. The check below compares the current state to that baseline. Walk through the session fully before completing the check.

> **NOTICE TODAY:**
> During the session, pay specific attention to the joints that were most symptomatic on Day 1. Compare their current experience to the morning of Day 1 as honestly as possible.

> **PROGRESS CHECK**
> *Two weeks of daily practice. Compare to your Week 1 results. Note any changes.*
>
> Morning stiffness rating this week: compare to your three-day pre-program average. a) Lower b) About the same c) Variable day to day
> Ward Off balance hold on the weaker side: compare to Day 1. a) Noticeably more stable b) Slightly more stable c) About the same
> Which joints feel most improved by the practice so far?   Which joints still feel most symptomatic?   Has morning stiffness onset changed? (When does it appear and how long does it last)
>
> Week Three adds four more forms and explicitly addresses mental clarity. Sessions increase to fifteen minutes. The cognitive engagement of the practice deepens significantly this week.

Knees, Hips, and Shoulders Getting Their Turn

Week Two is structured so that each of the three major joint areas receives specific attention in the new forms. White Crane targets the hip stabilizers and the shoulder superior arc. Repulse the Monkey provides sequential hip loading for both joints alternately. The hip joint responds to this week's specific sequence with measurable improvements in morning stiffness that typically appear between Day 12 and Day 14. If the improvement has not yet appeared by Day 14, it will typically do so in Week Three as the cumulative effect compounds.

Week 3 – Sharpen the Mind

Week Three adds Roll Back and Press, Fair Lady Works the Shuttles, and Golden Rooster Stands on One Leg to the sequence. All seven forms are now in the daily sequence. Sessions are fifteen minutes. The week's theme is explicit: mental clarity.

The cognitive engagement of this week is substantially higher than the previous two. Three new forms, each requiring its own motor program, are added simultaneously. The working memory is managing nine distinct form sequences by the end of this week. This is a genuine executive function load. The coaching notes in this week address the cognitive dimension directly: what mental clarity feels like when it begins to improve, how to notice the difference in attention quality between the start and end of a session.

What You Might Feel This Week
- A return of the cognitive tiredness from Week One as three new forms are added. This is normal and resolves within two to three sessions.
- Golden Rooster is the form that most commonly reveals the proprioceptive progress of the first two weeks. Many people find it measurably more stable than expected.
- Some people notice improved attention in non-practice contexts during this week: sharper focus during conversations, faster word retrieval, more present through ordinarily distracting tasks. This is the practice transferring.

Your Win This Week: Notice one specific improvement in mental clarity or attention quality outside of the practice sessions. Name it precisely.

Day 15 – Three New Forms

SESSION AT A GLANCE
15 minutes | Forms: All seven (Opening, Ward Off, Roll Back and Press, White Crane, Repulse, Fair Lady, Golden Rooster, Closing and Return) | Low-energy option: Opening Form, Ward Off, White Crane, Closing and Return, 5 mins

Liuhe's Note:
Three new forms. Read through each one before the session. Practice them separately before attempting the full sequence. The full sequence can wait until Day 16 or 17. Today is for learning, not completion.

NOTICE TODAY:
Golden Rooster: on the first attempt, how many seconds can you hold the single-leg position without gripping the chair? Record it. This is the beginning of a specific measurement.

Day 16 – The Full Sequence

SESSION AT A GLANCE
15 minutes | All seven forms in sequence | Focus: transitions between all seven | Low-energy option: Opening Form, Roll Back and Press, Closing and Return, 5 minutes

Liuhe's Note:
Attempt the full sequence today. Expect it to be imperfect. The quality of the forms will be lower than the three-form sequence of Week One. This is the correct response: new complexity demands new attention. Imperfect completion is the target, not perfect performance of a shortened sequence.

NOTICE TODAY:
Notice which of the new forms requires the most conscious attention to execute. That form is where the most cognitive work is happening this week.

Day 17 – The Mind Inside Golden Rooster

SESSION AT A GLANCE
15 minutes | All seven forms | Focus: cognitive engagement specifically in Golden Rooster | Low-energy option: Opening Form, Golden Rooster with chair support, Closing and Return, 5 minutes

Liuhe's Note:

Golden Rooster is this program's most demanding form for balance and for attention simultaneously. During today's holds, count the seconds aloud or silently. The counting is not to track time. It is to give the prefrontal cortex a specific task that prevents balance-disrupting mental chatter. Notice whether the hold is more stable when counting than when not.

NOTICE TODAY:
What kind of thinking disrupts the Golden Rooster hold most reliably? Noticing the content of the thoughts that break the balance reveals something about how attention and balance interact in your specific nervous system.

Day 18 – Rest

REST DAY
No formal practice session today. Rest is part of the program.

Liuhe's Note:
This rest day arrives at the midpoint of Week Three when the cognitive load of three new forms is highest. Mental tiredness at this stage is a sign of genuine learning, not weakness. Recovery is what converts that effort into retained skill.

Day 19 – Focus and Coordination

SESSION AT A GLANCE
15 minutes | All seven forms | Focus: bilateral coordination in Repulse and Fair Lady | Low-energy option: Opening Form, Ward Off, Fair Lady, Closing and Return, 5 minutes

Liuhe's Note:
The two forms that demand the most bilateral coordination are Repulse the Monkey and Fair Lady Works the Shuttles. In Repulse, both limbs move simultaneously in opposite patterns. In Fair Lady, the turning body and the rising arm must coordinate. Today, bring specific attention to the coordination quality of both forms. Coordination precision is a direct measure of prefrontal executive function.

NOTICE TODAY:
Has the bilateral coordination of Repulse the Monkey improved since Day 8? Describe the difference precisely. Vague impressions are less useful than specific comparisons.

Day 20 – The Mind-Body Shift

SESSION AT A GLANCE
15 minutes | All seven forms | Focus: allowing the forms to run with less conscious management | Low-energy option: Opening Form, White Crane, Closing and Return, 5 minutes

Liuhe's Note:
Today's instruction is to perform the sequence with less conscious management of each step. Allow the forms to run from the motor programs the brain has been building. Intervene only when something is genuinely wrong. The transition from conscious learning to fluent execution is what this day is testing. Some forms will run more fluently than others. That difference is information about where the motor programs are fully built.

NOTICE TODAY:
Which forms can now run with minimal conscious tracking? Which still require active attention? The list of fluent forms is longer than it was on Day 15. Count them.

PROGRESS CHECK
Three weeks complete. Compare your experience this week against your Week 2 check results.
BALANCE: Single-leg balance hold on your weaker side this week: compare to your Week Two check. a) Noticeably longer b) Slightly longer c) About the same
JOINT PAIN: Morning stiffness this week compared to your Week Two check: a) Lower b) About the same c) Variable
MENTAL CLARITY: Has the quality of your attention during the forms improved compared to Week Two? a) Yes, the forms feel more automatic b) Some forms, not all c) About the same
MENTAL CLARITY (DAILY LIFE): Has anything changed in your thinking, focus, or word retrieval outside of the practice sessions this week? a) Yes, specifically: b) Not yet measurable
BALANCE (FLUENCY): Which of the nine forms now flows without conscious tracking?

Week Four adds the Balance Builders after each session and extends sessions to 15–20 minutes. No new forms are introduced. This week deepens what has been built and tests how far the improvements have transferred into your daily life.

Day 21 – Rest Day

REST DAY

No formal practice session today. Rest is part of the program.

Liuhe's Note:
Three weeks complete. Today is a full rest day. The Week Three Progress Check is at the end of Day 20 above. Complete it there if you have not already. Use today to rest, reflect on what the forms have built, and read the section below.

Focus, Coordination, and the Mind-Body Shift

The mental clarity that Week Three addresses is not a vague feeling of wellness. It is a specific change in the availability and quality of attention. People who experience it during this week consistently describe it in the same terms: tasks that required effort last week feel like less effort now. The working memory has more headroom. The attention has more range. Word retrieval is faster. These are not coincidences. They are the downstream effects of three weeks of daily cortisol reduction and prefrontal cortex activation through the form sequences.

Week 4 – Stand Tall, Stay Sharp

Week Four adds the Balance Builders to the end of each session and extends the session to fifteen to twenty minutes. No new forms are introduced. This week is about deepening what has been built, not expanding it. The sequence now runs from Opening Form through Closing and Return, with the four Balance Builders following before the Closing and Return.

The final progress check at Day 28 completes the record that began with the Chapter Three self-assessment. By Day 28, most people who have completed the program consistently have measurable improvements in all three baseline areas. The check makes those improvements specific and legible, which is what makes them durable.

What You Might Feel This Week
- The Balance Builders will add a noticeable demand to the sessions, particularly Golden Rooster Stands on One Leg and Single-Leg Reach. By Day 26 the additional demand will feel routine.
- The full sequence plus Balance Builders may feel like a lot to hold in attention. It becomes less effortful by the third session of the week.
- Some people notice that the practice is beginning to feel like something they want to do rather than something they are doing. This shift in motivation is a signal that the practice has become genuinely established.

Your Win This Week: Complete every session with all nine forms and all four Balance Builders. Miss nothing this week.

Day 22 – Adding the Balance Builders

SESSION AT A GLANCE
15-20 minutes | All nine forms, then all four Balance Builders, then Closing and Return | Low-energy option: Five forms only, no Balance Builders, 5 mins

Liuhe's Note:
The Balance Builders follow the nine forms and come before the final Closing and Return. Perform them in order: Tandem Stand, Heel Raise with Eyes Closed, Lateral Weight Shift, Single-Leg Reach. Read through each one in Chapter Four before this session.

NOTICE TODAY:
Balance: during the Tandem Stand, notice whether the heel-to-toe balance feels different on the two foot arrangements. The less stable arrangement is the one that benefits most from the practice.

Day 23 – Joints at Full Sequence

SESSION AT A GLANCE
15-20 minutes | Full sequence with Balance Builders | Focus: joint experience through the complete session | Low-energy option: Opening Form, White Crane, one Balance Builder, Closing and Return, 5 minutes

Liuhe's Note:
Today the full sequence including Balance Builders is the practice. Bring attention specifically to the joints through the session. How do they feel at the beginning of Opening Form? How do they feel at the end of the Balance Builders? The difference is the session's joint effect in real time.

NOTICE TODAY:
Joint: which joint feels most improved during today's full sequence compared to the first week? Name the joint and describe the specific change in as few words as possible.

Day 24 – Mind Through the Full Sequence

SESSION AT A GLANCE
15-20 minutes | Full sequence with Balance Builders | Focus: attention quality through the complete 20 minutes | Low-energy option: Opening Form, Ward Off, Closing and Return with five breath cycles, 5 minutes

Liuhe's Note:
The cognitive demand of the complete sequence plus Balance Builders is the highest it has been in the program. Notice whether attention is maintained through the full duration or whether it drifts in the later forms. The point in the sequence where attention first drifts is the point where the prefrontal resources are most depleted. Over further weeks of practice, this point moves later.

NOTICE TODAY:
Clarity: after the full session and Closing and Return, rate the clarity of thinking on a scale of one to five compared to this morning before the session. Note the number. Compare it to how you would have rated it before Day 1.

Day 25 – Rest

REST DAY
No formal practice session today. Rest is part of the program.

Liuhe's Note:
The first rest day of Week Four protects the balance and fluency gains of the week so far. By this point the full sequence should feel more automatic. That automaticity consolidates during recovery, not during additional practice volume.

Day 26 – The Practice That Belongs to You

SESSION AT A GLANCE
15-20 minutes | Full sequence with Balance Builders | Focus: attending to what the practice feels like from inside | Low-energy option: Opening Form, favorite two forms, Closing and Return, 5 minutes

Liuhe's Note:
Two sessions remain. Today's session has one simple instruction: attend to what the practice feels like from inside your body, not from outside it. Not how the forms look or whether they

are correct. What the weight feels like moving through the foot. What the breath feels like coordinating with the arms. What the stillness of Closing and Return feels like at the end. This is how the practice becomes yours rather than mine.

NOTICE TODAY:
What is one thing about this practice that you did not expect when you began on Day 1?

Day 27 – Rest

REST DAY
No formal practice session today. Rest is part of the program.

Liuhe's Note:
The final rest day of the program. Tomorrow is Day 28 and the final progress check. Arriving there with some freshness produces a more accurate and more encouraging review. Rest fully today.

Day 28 – Full Body and Mind Review

SESSION AT A GLANCE
15-20 minutes | Full sequence with Balance Builders | Closing: complete the Day 28 progress check after the session | Low-energy option: Opening Form, Ward Off, Closing and Return, 5 minutes

Liuhe's Note:
Twenty-eight days. Perform the full session first. Close with five breath cycles. Then complete the check below. The check is the record. The practice is what matters.

NOTICE TODAY:
Walk through the session with the Day 1 assessment in mind. Compare what was true on Day 1 to what is true today, for each of the three baselines, inside the session itself.

PROGRESS CHECK
Day 28. The final check. Return to the Chapter Three baselines and all intermediate progress check records. Compare each one honestly.

Single-leg balance hold today: left (   ) sec, right (   ) sec. Chapter Three baseline: left (   ) sec, right (   ) sec.
Joint stiffness morning rating today (1-5):   . Chapter Three - three-day average: . a) Improved b) Same c) Variable

Three-minute attention test: attention lapses today: . Chapter Three baseline: .
Golden Rooster hold duration today vs Day 15 vs Day 21: Day 15:   sec. Day 21:   sec.
Today: sec.
Which of the nine forms do you feel most confident in?
Name one specific way your daily life is different because of this practice:

Chapter Eight addresses how to read this review honestly and what to do next. Read it before
deciding anything about the future of the practice.

End of Week Four: Full Body and Mind Review

The Day 28 review is not a test. It is the last measurement in a series that began before Day 1. The value of the measurement is not in whether the numbers are large. It is in the record of where the practice has moved each baseline over the course of twenty-eight days, and in the specific, named observation of one way daily life has changed. That observation is the independence outcome this program was designed to produce.

Whatever the review shows, the practice that produced the changes is available every morning, in ten to twenty minutes, in whatever space you have. Chapter Eight addresses the three honest questions this review raises and the three options for what comes next.

Chapter 6

Sleep, Rest, and the Recovery Loop

The three benefits this practice delivers are not completed during the session. They are initiated during the session and completed during sleep. This distinction is not a small one.

Why Recovery Is Half the Practice

There is a tendency, particularly among people beginning a new health practice, to believe that more is better and that rest is the absence of progress. In a practice designed around slow deliberate movement and neural adaptation, this belief is incorrect in a specific and important way.

The standing forms create conditions in the body and brain that adaptation then fulfills during rest. The proprioceptive training of Golden Rooster, for example, stimulates the ankle and hip mechanoreceptors to fire more precisely and more rapidly during the form. But the neural pathway changes that make this firing more reliable in tomorrow's session, and in the balance demands of ordinary daily life, are written during the deep sleep that follows the practice day. The practice opens the adaptation window. Sleep closes it productively.

The same principle applies to joint health. The synovial fluid circulation that the forms stimulate distributes nutrients through the cartilage during the session. But the anti-inflammatory cytokines that repair the micro-inflammatory processes in the joint tissue are released primarily during deep sleep, particularly in the first half of the night when slow-wave sleep is most concentrated. A night of disrupted or shortened sleep following a practice session reduces the repair that the session made possible.

And for mental clarity: the cortisol reduction that the breath coordination of the forms produces creates a more favorable environment for memory consolidation. But the actual consolidation of what was learned during the session, the form sequences, the proprioceptive patterns, the breath timing, happens during REM sleep. This is why a well-slept night after a practice session produces more fluent forms the following morning than a poorly slept one, even though no practice happened overnight.

Rest days are part of the same system. The two scheduled rest days in this program are not concessions to limitation. They are required components of the adaptation process. The body and nervous system that are asked to adapt every day without recovery do not adapt as efficiently as those given scheduled recovery windows. The rest days are where the Week One proprioceptive gains consolidate, where the Week Two joint lubrication improvements compound, and where the Week Three cognitive changes become baseline rather than session-specific.

This is why the instruction in Chapter Five not to substitute practice sessions for rest days is not arbitrary. A practitioner who replaces Day 4's rest with an extra session is not being more dedicated. They are interrupting the consolidation that the Day 1 through 3 sessions created. The extra session produces less benefit than the rest would have, and the following week begins from a less consolidated foundation. Rest days are not passive. They are active recovery, and they are as important to the three-benefit outcome as the practice sessions themselves.

How Tai Chi Changes Sleep Quality After 60

Poor sleep and aging are not the same thing, although they frequently coincide. The sleep architecture changes that occur after sixty, reduced slow-wave sleep, earlier wake times, more frequent nighttime awakenings, are driven partly by the same cortisol dysregulation that contributes to joint stiffness and cognitive fog during the day. Addressing the cortisol is the lever that influences all three.

Consistent standing Tai Chi practice reduces diurnal cortisol through two mechanisms. The first is the parasympathetic activation of the breath coordination during the session, which produces an acute cortisol drop that typically lasts two to three hours after the session. The second is the cumulative effect of weeks of daily parasympathetic activation, which shifts the baseline cortisol level downward over time. A lower baseline cortisol level improves sleep architecture at night by reducing the hyperarousal that disrupts slow-wave sleep initiation and maintenance.

The specific sleep improvements that practitioners report, typically beginning in Week Two, include faster sleep onset, fewer nighttime awakenings, more settled sleep in the first half of the night, and a morning quality of alertness that is qualitatively different from pre-practice mornings. These reports are consistent with the documented effects of regular Tai Chi practice on cortisol and sleep architecture in older adult populations. The improvements are not guaranteed or uniform, but they are common and they are mechanistically explained.

Morning practice is specifically advantageous for sleep quality. A morning session produces a cortisol drop in the morning hours and allows the baseline to remain lower through the afternoon and evening, which is precisely when it needs to be low enough to allow sleep initiation. Evening practice, while beneficial in other ways, can produce a mild activation effect in some individuals that delays sleep onset. Morning practice avoids this and positions the cortisol reduction where it is most useful for the sleep that follows.

The improvement in sleep quality that most practitioners report beginning in Week Two is not uniform. Some people notice it first as faster sleep onset: they are asleep within ten minutes rather than the thirty or forty minutes of pre-program nights. Others notice it as fewer awakenings: they sleep through the hours that previously involved two or three trips to consciousness. Still others notice it as a difference in the quality of morning alertness rather than the architecture of the sleep itself: they wake feeling more restored. All of these are expressions of the same underlying change, which is the downward shift in baseline cortisol that the daily practice produces. The specific form the improvement takes is individual. The mechanism is consistent.

What Happens to Joints During Sleep

The joint capsule is an immunologically active environment. During waking hours, the physical demands placed on the joints, combined with the inflammatory products of normal cellular metabolism, create a mild pro-inflammatory environment in the joint tissue. The body's anti-inflammatory systems manage this continuously during the day. During sleep, the metabolic demand on the joints drops significantly, and the anti-inflammatory cytokines, particularly interleukin-10 and transforming growth factor-beta, are released in their highest concentrations to repair the accumulated inflammation of the day.

When sleep is poor, this nightly repair is incomplete. The inflammatory accumulation from the previous day is not fully resolved before the next day's demands begin. Over weeks, this incomplete clearance compounds into a higher baseline inflammatory state in the joint. This is the mechanism behind the observation that people with chronic sleep problems have higher rates of joint pain severity than those who sleep well, independent of structural differences in the joints themselves.

Cartilage repair also depends on overnight conditions. The growth hormone that stimulates cartilage cell activity and matrix synthesis is released in its largest pulse during the first period of slow-wave sleep. Poor slow-wave sleep means less growth hormone and slower cartilage maintenance. The Tai Chi practice that improves slow-wave sleep through cortisol reduction is therefore contributing to cartilage maintenance through an indirect pathway that most practitioners are unaware of: better practice leads to better sleep leads to better joint repair overnight.

The practical implication is that the quality of sleep on practice-day nights matters to the joint outcome of this program as much as the quality of the practice session itself. A session followed by eight hours of deep, restorative sleep produces more joint benefit than the same session followed by five hours of fragmented sleep. This is not a reason to add sleep to the list of things to manage anxiously. It is a reason to recognize that everything in this system is connected, and that the habits described later in this chapter support not just the cognitive and balance benefits but the joint repair that happens overnight.

What Happens to Balance During Rest

The proprioceptive improvements that the standing forms produce are neural changes: the mechanoreceptors in the ankle, knee, and hip joints are sending more reliable signals, the neural pathways carrying those signals are more efficient, and the brain regions processing the signals are responding more rapidly. These changes are initiated by the practice and consolidated during sleep through a process called motor memory consolidation.

Motor memory consolidation during sleep is not metaphorical. The hippocampus and cerebellum replay and strengthen the motor sequences practiced during waking hours during the slow-wave and REM sleep periods that follow. The proprioceptive patterns that were trained during the session become more deeply encoded as the night progresses. A person who practiced Golden Rooster for the first time on Day 15 and slept well afterward will demonstrate measurably better single-leg balance in Day 16's session than someone who practiced the same form but slept poorly.

The vestibular system follows the same consolidation pattern. The head-movement forms that challenge the vestibular calibration become more fluent overnight. The balance responses that were effortful and conscious during the session become more automatic and less consciously managed in subsequent sessions. This automaticity is the target: a balance system that responds below the level of conscious attention is faster and more reliable than one that requires conscious management of every perturbation.

What Happens to Mental Clarity During Sleep

The prefrontal cortex, the region most responsible for the clear thinking this practice supports, is also the region most dependent on sleep for its overnight recovery. The metabolic byproducts of a day of cognitive work are cleared from the prefrontal cortex during sleep through the glymphatic system, a waste-clearance mechanism that operates primarily during slow-wave sleep. When slow-wave sleep is shortened or disrupted, this clearance is incomplete. The prefrontal cortex begins the following day carrying a higher metabolic load, which manifests as the cognitive heaviness and reduced processing speed that many older adults experience on mornings after poor sleep.

The form sequences learned during the practice session are processed overnight in the hippocampus and transferred into longer-term procedural memory. This is why forms that felt difficult and required active conscious management on Day 1 feel progressively more automatic by Day 7: seven nights of consolidation have moved the motor program from effortful working memory into fluent procedural storage. The forms become more available to conscious attention once the mechanical sequence is automated, which is why Week Three's focus on mental clarity becomes possible only after two weeks of form learning have been consolidated overnight.

The Morning Window – Your Most Powerful 10 Minutes

The morning window, the period of approximately thirty to sixty minutes after waking, is the optimal time for this practice for reasons that extend beyond habit and convenience.

The cortisol awakening response, the physiological spike in cortisol that occurs in the first thirty minutes after waking, is at its peak during this window. This spike serves a biological purpose: it mobilizes energy, primes the immune system, and prepares the body for the day's demands. Practicing at the tail end of this spike, as it is naturally declining, means the practice's parasympathetic activation and cortisol-lowering mechanism are working with the cortisol's natural trajectory rather than against an already declining curve. The result is a more pronounced and more sustained cortisol reduction than a later-day session produces.

The morning practice also positions the day's cortisol trajectory favorably. A lower cortisol level established in the morning persists through the afternoon and evening, supporting clearer thinking through the working hours and lower arousal through the evening hours that support sleep. The ten minutes of morning practice has a disproportionate influence on the hormonal environment of the entire day.

Practically: do the Pre-Practice Joint Preparation sequence from Chapter Three before beginning the forms. The joints are at their stiffest in the morning and need two to three minutes of gentle mobilization before the weight-shifting demands of the forms are appropriate. The preparation sequence addresses exactly the joint state the morning presents. After it, the forms begin in a more favorable mechanical environment and the session produces more joint benefit than it would without the preparation. This preparation also gives the nervous system a transitional period between sleeping and moving, which reduces the cortisol spike that abrupt morning physical activity can trigger in some individuals.

Chapter 7

Living in a Sharper, Steadier Body

The forms are a daily practice. The benefits are a continuous state. This chapter is about the gap between the two: how the ten minutes of morning practice becomes a changed relationship with the body and mind throughout the rest of the day.

Applying the Forms to Daily Life At Home

The standing forms train specific capacities: single-leg balance, deliberate weight transfer, coordinated breath, sequential attention. These capacities do not switch off when the session ends. They transfer into the ordinary movements of the day in proportion to how well the forms have been learned and how consistently the practice has been maintained.

Getting up from a chair is the movement that practitioners most frequently identify as changed by this practice. Rising from seated to standing is a single-leg loading event: the weight transfers from the seat to the feet, the quadriceps extend the knees, and for a brief moment the body is managing a significant loading force through the hip and knee joints before the standing position is fully established. The same quadriceps that the Ward Off and Golden Rooster forms have been strengthening through slow deliberate loading manage this transition. People who have practiced for four weeks consistently report that rising from a chair feels more controlled, requires less push from the armrests, and produces less knee discomfort than it did before the program.

Navigating stairs involves single-leg loading demands even more concentrated than Ward Off. Each step up requires the leading leg to extend from a bent knee under the full body weight. Each step down requires the trailing leg to control the body's descent through an eccentric quadriceps contraction. The balance training of Golden Rooster and White Crane provides the hip stability that prevents the pelvis from tilting sideways during each stair step, which is one of the most common mechanical contributors to stair-related falls. People who have completed this program consistently report more confidence on stairs, particularly on descent, where the eccentric loading demand is highest.

Standing in a queue is a balance challenge that most people do not recognize as one until their balance system is under stress. Standing still for several minutes on a hard surface, particularly in footwear that reduces ground feel, is a sustained proprioceptive demand. The mechanoreceptors are continuously reporting small postural drift and requesting small corrections. After four weeks of daily proprioceptive training through the forms, this sustained standing demand is managed with less effort and less visible sway than before the practice.

Reaching, Bending, and Lifting Without Pain

Three categories of household movement are most commonly associated with joint pain and fall risk in older adults: reaching overhead for stored objects, bending to retrieve things from low surfaces, and lifting objects that carry asymmetric weight. Each transfers directly from the forms.

Overhead reaching engages the shoulder in its superior arc, the same movement that Fair Lady Works the Shuttles trains deliberately. After several weeks of practice, the rotator cuff muscles that stabilize the shoulder during overhead reach are stronger and more coordinately active than before. The reach itself is more controlled and produces less impingement pain in the superior joint space. People who previously avoided overhead reaching because of shoulder discomfort frequently find it more manageable after four to six weeks of consistent Fair Lady practice.

The thoracic rotation that Fair Lady also requires transfers to the rotational demands of reaching sideways and across the body, movements that are involved in every kitchen and household task. The thoracic spine that was stiff and resistant to rotation in Week One, producing compensatory lumbar rotation and the resulting lower back discomfort, is progressively more mobile by Week Four. This increased thoracic rotation range means that the lower back is no longer required to compensate for thoracic restriction during ordinary reaching and turning movements. The lower back discomfort that accompanied these movements often reduces as a secondary benefit of the shoulder and thoracic mobility work, even though the lower back was never the primary target.

Bending to retrieve objects from low surfaces involves hip hinge mechanics: the torso lowers while the hips flex and the lumbar spine maintains its neutral curve. The neutral spine instruction that runs through all nine forms, the foundational posture requirement of the practice, directly trains the lumbar and thoracic muscles that hold the spine in its functional position during a bend. The hip flexor flexibility that the forms build reduces the compression on the posterior lumbar discs during the bend. Practitioners report fewer episodes of low back pain from bending tasks after four weeks of consistent practice.

Lifting with asymmetric load, carrying a shopping bag in one hand, transfers from the Wave Step balance builder and the single-leg forms. An asymmetric carry shifts the body's center of mass toward the loaded side and requires the hip stabilizers of the opposite side to produce a sustained corrective force. The gluteus medius on the unloaded side that the Lateral Weight Shift balance builder specifically trains is the primary muscle managing this correction. Stronger hip stabilizers produce a steadier carry with less spinal tilt and less fatigue through the lower back and hip.

Mental Sharpness Beyond the Practice

The cognitive improvements from this practice extend beyond the session in three specific ways that practitioners most reliably report.

The first is attention stability: the ability to maintain focus on a single task through distractions that would previously have pulled it away. This is the direct transfer of the sustained attention that the form sequences require. Holding the sequence in mind while managing breath and balance trains the executive attention network of the prefrontal cortex. After weeks of daily training, this network is more capable in ordinary cognitive tasks. The person who previously lost their train of thought during a conversation when a phone notification appeared finds the distraction more manageable. The person who previously had to reread a paragraph three times to retain it finds it settling on the first reading.

The second is word retrieval: the ability to access the word or name that felt stuck on the tip of the tongue before the practice. Word retrieval is primarily a hippocampal function and is one of the cognitive processes most sensitive to cortisol. The cortisol reduction that this practice produces over weeks improves hippocampal function directly, and the improvement in word retrieval is often the cognitive change that practitioners notice and remark on most specifically.

The third is processing speed: the rapidity with which the brain handles a sequence of incoming information and generates an appropriate response. Processing speed declines with both age and elevated cortisol. Regular Tai Chi practice addresses both pathways: the age-related decline is slowed by the active engagement of multiple neural networks simultaneously during the forms, and the cortisol-related impairment is reduced by the practice's sustained cortisol-lowering effect.

A fourth cognitive benefit that practitioners less commonly anticipate is emotional regulation: the ability to respond to frustrating or stressful events with a measured rather than an automatic reaction. Emotional regulation is a prefrontal executive function, and like the other executive functions described above, it is strengthened by regular engagement and impaired by cortisol. The same prefrontal strengthening that improves attention and processing speed in this practice also improves the capacity to pause between provocation and response. This is not a personality change. It is a physiological change in the cortisol environment and the prefrontal capacity that operates within it. Practitioners who notice this change often describe it as feeling less reactive, less pulled into conflict, more able to let difficult things pass without the same internal cost they carried before.

Daily Habits That Lock In the Gains

Four daily habits support the three benefits of the practice in the hours between sessions. Each takes less than two minutes and each is derived directly from the form principles.

The first is the standing posture reset. At any point during the day when you notice yourself standing, apply the foundational posture of the Opening Form: feet shoulder-width, knees soft, spine long, shoulders relaxed, chin level. Hold it for three breath cycles. This two-minute posture reset reduces the cumulative spinal compression and hip flexor tension that prolonged standing with poor alignment creates, and it delivers a brief cortisol reduction through the breath coordination.

The second is the seated breath practice. When sitting for extended periods, particularly in front of screens, place both feet flat on the floor and complete five cycles of the Tai Chi breath: inhale for four counts, exhale for six counts. This brief parasympathetic activation counteracts the cortisol accumulation of sustained cognitive work and provides a reset for the prefrontal cortex that is measurable in the subsequent fifteen minutes of cognitive performance.

The third is the deliberate transition. When moving from one activity to another, particularly when rising from a chair, deliberately slow the movement to half speed and apply the weight-transfer awareness of the forms. This takes three to four seconds rather than the one second of a habitual transition, and it provides a brief proprioceptive training stimulus outside the formal session. Over the course of a day with multiple transitions, these accumulated three-second deliberate movements add a meaningful additional proprioceptive load to the system.

The fourth is the pre-sleep joint release. In the five minutes before sleep, while lying in bed, gently rotate both ankles in slow circles, flex and extend both knees, and roll both shoulders backward and forward. These micro-movements stimulate the synovial fluid circulation in the three joint areas the forms most directly address and position the joints in a more favorable biochemical state for the overnight repair that sleep initiates. The sequence takes less than three minutes and produces a measurable reduction in morning stiffness when practiced consistently.

The cumulative effect of all four daily habits, practiced alongside the morning session, is a body and mind that receive the benefits of the practice more continuously than the ten-minute session alone provides. The morning session creates the primary adaptation stimulus. The four habits extend and reinforce its effects through the hours that follow. Together they constitute not a program but a way of living in the body: attentive, deliberate, and kind to the specific systems that determine how the day feels from the inside.

The habits also serve as anchors for the attention quality that the forms develop. Each of the four takes less than three minutes. Each requires a brief but genuine shift from automatic behavior to deliberate awareness. The standing posture reset, the seated breath, the deliberate transition, the pre-sleep joint release: none of them are difficult. All of them are easily forgotten. The practitioner who maintains all four alongside the daily session is practicing not just the forms but the orientation toward the body that the forms are designed to cultivate.

Chapter 8

After Day 28

Day 28 is not an ending. It is the first day that the practice has a history long enough to be honestly evaluated. This chapter helps with that evaluation.

Three Honest Questions to Ask Yourself

The Day 28 progress check at the end of Chapter Five produced specific data: single-leg balance hold times, a joint stiffness rating, an attention lapse count, and a named daily life change. Before deciding what comes next, sit with the following three questions. Answer them specifically rather than generally. Specific answers are the useful ones.

The first question is: what actually changed? Compare the three Chapter Three baselines to the Day 28 measurements and name the changes that are real, that are specific, and that you would be comfortable describing to someone else in precise terms. Not 'I feel better' but 'My single-leg balance hold on the right side increased from four seconds to eighteen seconds.' Not 'My joints are less stiff' but 'Morning stiffness in my left knee now resolves within ten minutes rather than forty.' The precision matters because it is what allows you to track continued progress beyond Day 28 and to recognize when the practice has produced a genuine plateau that merits a program change.

The second question is: what did not change that you expected to change? Honest disappointment is more useful than vague satisfaction. If joint pain in a specific location did not improve despite four weeks of daily practice, that is important information. It may mean the joint requires medical evaluation rather than further exercise. It may mean the form modifications needed to protect that joint were not applied consistently. It may mean the form sequence that most directly addresses that joint was not practiced with sufficient attention. Identifying which of these is most likely is the first step toward addressing it.

The third question is: what surprised you? The surprise answers are often the most informative. People who expected balance improvement and got it are not surprised. People who expected balance improvement, got it, and also found that word retrieval improved and sleep deepened have learned something about their own physiology that the expectation did not predict. The surprises are where the individual response to the practice is most clearly visible, and they tend to point toward the benefits that will be most durable and most personally meaningful in the continued practice.

When to Progress, When to Repeat, When to Rest

Three trajectories are available after Day 28, and each is appropriate for different outcomes.

Progress means extending the practice: longer sessions, more challenging balance demands, the introduction of outdoor walking with the proprioceptive demands of uneven terrain, or the addition of more advanced Tai Chi sequences beyond the nine forms of this program. Progression is appropriate when the Day 28 review shows clear improvement across all three benefit areas and when the nine forms flow with sufficient fluency that the motor management no longer requires heavy conscious attention. In practice, people who complete Week Four with consistent daily sessions and clear progress checks in all three areas are ready to progress.

Repeat means running the twenty-eight-day program a second time from Week One. Repetition is appropriate when the Day 28 review shows improvement in one or two of the three benefit areas but incomplete improvement in the third, or when the nine forms arc not yet fluent enough to allow the attention to move above the level of motor management. The second run of the program produces a qualitatively different experience from the first: the forms are familiar, the learning load is lower, and the attention that was consumed by form acquisition in the first run can now be directed toward the depth of the proprioceptive feedback, the precision of the breath timing, and the specific sensation of the balance mechanisms the forms are training. Most people find the second run more rewarding than the first.

Rest is appropriate when the Day 28 review reveals that a specific condition needs medical evaluation: joint pain that has not responded to four weeks of gentle daily practice, a balance issue that has worsened rather than improved, or cognitive symptoms that feel more prominent than before the program began. These are rare outcomes and they do not indicate that the program failed. They indicate that the condition requires a level of support beyond what a home movement practice can provide, and that the appropriate next step is professional evaluation rather than continued self-directed practice.

Joint Pain That Didn't Shift – What to Do Next

If joint pain in a specific location is unchanged or worsened after four weeks of this program, three possibilities deserve consideration.

The first possibility is structural: the joint has a degree of damage that deliberate gentle movement cannot address without clinical support. Moderate to severe osteoarthritis with significant cartilage loss, joint space narrowing visible on imaging, or a prior injury that altered the joint's mechanical axis are all conditions in which this program may need to be a supplement to rather than a replacement for clinical management. A physiotherapist or orthopedic specialist can assess the specific joint and advise on whether the forms are appropriate to continue, with modifications, alongside clinical treatment.

The second possibility is technical: the form modifications for that specific joint were not applied, or were applied inconsistently. The knee guidance in Chapter Three, for example, describes specific techniques for managing knee load during the forms. If these were not used, or if the session pace was too high for the available knee range of motion, the forms may have been adding load rather than providing relief. Reviewing the relevant Chapter Three guidance for that joint and applying it rigorously to a second program run often resolves pain that did not shift in the first.

The third possibility is systemic: the joint pain is being driven by a cortisol environment that four weeks of practice has not yet lowered sufficiently to produce a measurable anti-inflammatory effect. This is most likely in individuals with significant ongoing life stress, poor sleep quality, or a medical condition that elevates cortisol independently of the practice. In these cases, addressing the systemic drivers directly, through sleep intervention, stress management, or medical management of the underlying condition, alongside the continued Tai Chi practice, is the appropriate response. Four weeks is a beginning for some conditions, and not a completion for them.

Turning 28 Days Into a Lifelong Rhythm

The factor that determines whether this practice becomes a permanent feature of life or a completed program is not motivation. Motivation is unreliable and fluctuates with mood, circumstance, and the availability of other demands. The factor is structure: the degree to which the practice has been embedded in a daily routine that removes the need for a motivational decision each morning.

Practices that require a decision each time they occur are practices that are eventually skipped when the decision is made under conditions of fatigue, social demand, or competing priority. Practices that are embedded in a fixed-time, fixed-location routine that is already established do not require a decision. They simply occur, the way teeth-brushing occurs, because the routine produces the behavior without deliberate effort.

The structure that most reliably embeds this practice is: a fixed time each morning (within thirty minutes of the usual waking time), a fixed space (the same area of the same room), and a fixed sequence start (the Pre-Practice Joint Preparation from Chapter Three before Opening Form). These three fixed elements create the environmental cue chain that habits depend on. When all three are consistent, the practice becomes the default behavior of the morning rather than something that must be chosen.

What this practice gives back over years is not dramatic. It is the accumulation of small differences that compound: the fall that did not happen, the morning that was not lost to stiffness, the word that was retrieved rather than lost, the staircase that was climbed rather than avoided. These are not measurable in a single morning. They are the record of a practice that showed up consistently, across seasons and circumstances, for as long as the person chose to continue. That choice, made freshly each morning and made easier by the structure that removes the decision, is what the practice ultimately is.

There will be weeks when the practice does not happen every day. Illness, travel, disruption to the routine, all interrupt even the best-embedded habits. The appropriate response to an interrupted week is not to treat it as a failure and abandon the structure. It is to return to Day 1 of the routine: same time, same space, same opening sequence, on the first available morning. The practice does not judge the gap. It simply resumes. And the body and mind that took four weeks to build the first adaptation do not require another four weeks to restore it.

After a week away, most people find the forms return within two to three sessions. The foundation is still there.

Did You Find This Book Quite Helpful?

If it did, then that's worth something and deserves a place on Amazon.

Leaving a review takes two minutes and nothing else. For a book like this one, written without a publisher's marketing team or advertising spend, that two minutes is how it finds its next reader. It is how someone's daughter spots it while looking for something to give her mother. It is how this work keeps going. Two sentences is all it needs.

Search ***Standing Tai Chi for Seniors Over 60 by Liuhe Chen*** on Amazon. One or two honest sentences is all it takes.

Thank you for reading. It was an honor to take this trip with you.

Conclusion

What Changed in Your Body

The balance system you have now is not the same one you had on Day 1. The mechanoreceptors in your ankles and hips have been trained daily for four weeks. The neural pathways carrying their signals are more active and more efficient than they were. The single-leg hold that was uncertain or impossible on Day 1 is measurable in seconds on Day 28. This is a structural neural change, not a temporary improvement. It persists with continued practice and continues to develop. The fall that does not happen because the foot reads the ground before the weight follows it is not a dramatic event. It is a quiet outcome of this work.

The joints that moved through the forms each morning have been receiving synovial fluid circulation that they were not receiving before. The cartilage is better nourished. The morning stiffness that marked your pre-program mornings has reduced, if not disappeared. The cortisol that was driving inflammation in the joint tissue has been lower, consistently, for four weeks. These changes are real and they are the direct consequence of ten deliberate minutes each morning.

What Changed in Your Mind

The prefrontal cortex that managed the form sequences each morning is more capable than it was before the program. The sustained attention that the forms required has strengthened the executive attention networks that serve clear thinking throughout the day. The cortisol reduction has cleared the glucocorticoid load from the hippocampus that was impairing memory consolidation. The sleep that has improved over the course of the program has given the brain the overnight clearance and consolidation it needs to begin each day more fully restored than before.

These are not metaphors. They are physiological outcomes of a specific practice applied consistently over a sufficient duration. The mind that feels clearer, that retrieves words more readily, that holds attention through conversations and tasks with less effort, is a mind that has been trained by the same ten minutes that trained the balance and the joints. One practice, three benefits, because the practice was always addressing one interconnected system.

A Final Word from the Author

The word stillness in the title of this conclusion does not mean absence of movement. It means the quality of steadiness that a practiced body and a practiced mind produce: the ability to stand in a moment of uncertainty without the fear that uncertainty requires flight, to be present in the body without bracing against it, to think clearly without the cortisol fog that passes for ordinary aging in a life without deliberate practice.

You showed up for ten minutes each morning for twenty-eight days. You stood in your practice space and paid attention to how you move. That is not a small thing. Most people never do it. Most people manage the decline that comes with sixty and seventy and eighty as if management were the only option available.

The option available here is different. It is not dramatic. It does not reverse the decades. But it moves the trajectory. The balance improves. The joints move more freely. The mind is more available. And each of these, compounding across the years that follow Day 28, produces a life that is larger in the ways that matter most: more places navigated, more mornings that begin well, more of the thinking that makes a person feel like themselves.

Keep the practice. It has always belonged to you. Day 28 simply made that clear.

About The Author

Liuhe Chen has practiced Tai Chi for over twenty years. Most of that time has been spent teaching older adults, many of whom had never tried anything like it before and were not sure their bodies were up to it.

Some came after a fall. Some came on doctor's advice. Some came because a friend dragged them along and they ended up staying. Whatever brought them through the door, most of them had one thing in common: they wanted to feel steadier, stronger, and more confident in their own body. That is what Liuhe has spent two decades helping people achieve.

The teaching has always been simple. No complicated moves. No pressure to keep up. Just gentle, steady practice that meets people where they are, whether that means sitting in a chair, moving slowly through joint pain, or starting from scratch after years of little activity. Liuhe has worked with people in their seventies, eighties, and beyond, and has seen again and again that age is not the obstacle most people assume it is.

This book grew out of all those years of working with real people in real situations. It is written for anyone who wants to move better, feel better, and age on their own terms.

Liuhe practices every morning, rain or shine, and still finds something new in it each time.

www.ingramcontent.com/pod-product-compliance
Lightning Source LLC
Chambersburg PA
CBHW081931120726
47997CB00010B/3111